MIDWIFERY ESSENTIALS

Infant Feeding

T0195474

For Elsevier
Content Strategist: Alison Taylor
Content Development Specialist: Veronika Watkins
Project Manager: Julie Taylor
Designer: Paula Catalano
Illustration: Amy Faith Heyden

VOLUME **5**

MIDWIFERY ESSENTIALS

Infant Feeding

Joyce Marshall, RN, RM, BSc (Hons), MPH, PhD, PGCAP, FHEA
Senior Lecturer, Department of Health Sciences, University of
Huddersfield, Huddersfield, UK

Helen Baston, BA(Hons), MMedSci, PhD, PGDipEd, ADM, RN, RM
Consultant Midwife Public Health; Sheffield Teaching Hospitals NHS
Foundation Trust, UK; Honorary Researcher/Lecturer, University of
Sheffield, UK; Honorary Lecturer, Sheffield Hallam University, UK

Jenny Hall, EdD, MSc, RN, RM, ADM, PGDip(HE), SFHEA
Senior Midwifery Lecturer, Bournemouth University, UK

ELSEVIER

Edinburgh London New York Oxford Philadelphia St Louis Sydney Toronto 2017

ELSEVIER

ISBN 978-0-7020-7101-0
e_ISBN 978-0-7020-7146-1

British Library Cataloguing in Publication Data
A catalogue record for this book is available from the British Library

Library of Congress Cataloging in Publication Data
A catalog record for this book is available from the Library of Congress

Notices
Knowledge and best practice in this field are constantly changing. As new research and experience broaden our understanding, changes in research methods, professional practices, or medical treatment may become necessary.

Practitioners and researchers must always rely on their own experience and knowledge in evaluating and using any information, methods, compounds, or experiments described herein. In using such information or methods they should be mindful of their own safety and the safety of others, including parties for whom they have a professional responsibility.

With respect to any drug or pharmaceutical products identified, readers are advised to check the most current information provided (i) on procedures featured or (ii) by the manufacturer of each product to be administered, to verify the recommended dose or formula, the method and duration of administration, and contraindications. It is the responsibility of practitioners, relying on their own experience and knowledge of their patients, to make diagnoses, to determine dosages and the best treatment for each individual patient, and to take all appropriate safety precautions.

To the fullest extent of the law, neither the Publisher nor the authors, contributors, or editors, assume any liability for any injury and/or damage to persons or property as a matter of products liability, negligence or otherwise, or from any use or operation of any methods, products, instructions, or ideas contained in the material herein.

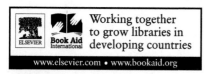

Working together
to grow libraries in
developing countries

www.elsevier.com • www.bookaid.org

your source for books,
journals and multimedia
in the health sciences

www.elsevierhealth.com

The
publisher's
policy is to use
paper manufactured
from sustainable forests

Printed in Great Britain
Last digit is the print number: 10 9 8 7 6 5 4 3

Contents

Preface

To contribute to the provision of sensitive, safe and effective maternity care for women and their families is a privilege. Childbirth is a life-changing event for women. Those around them and those who input into any aspect of pregnancy, labour, birth or the postnatal period can positively influence how this event is experienced and perceived. In order to achieve this, maternity carers continually need to reflect on the services they provide and strive to keep up to date with developments in clinical practice. They should endeavour to ensure that women are central to the decisions made and that real choices are offered and supported by skilled practitioners.

This book is the fifth volume in a series of texts based on the popular 'Midwifery Basics' series published in *The Practising Midwife* journal. The books have remained true to the original style of the articles and have been updated and expanded to create a user-friendly source of information. They are also intended to stimulate debate and require the reader both to reflect on their current practice, local policies and procedures and to challenge care that is not woman-centred. The use of scenarios enables the practitioner to understand the context of maternity care and explore their role in its safe and effective provision.

There are many dimensions to the provision of woman-centred care that practitioners need to consider and understand. To aid this process, a jigsaw model has been introduced, with the aim of encouraging the reader to explore maternity care from a wide range of perspectives. For example, how does a midwife obtain consent from a woman for a procedure, maintain a safe environment during the delivery of care and make the most of the opportunity to promote health? What are the professional and legal issues in relation to the procedure, and is this practice based on the best available evidence? Which members of the multi-professional team contribute to this aspect of care, and how is it influenced by the way care is organized? Each aspect of the jigsaw should be considered during the assessment, planning, implementation and evaluation of woman-centred maternity care.

Midwifery Essentials: Infant Feeding is a new addition to the series and is about the provision of safe and effective care to women and their babies. It reflects the focus of the UNICEF Baby Friendly Initiative Standards – supporting parents to develop close and loving relationships with their infants. It comprises 12 chapters, each written to stand alone or to be read in succession. The introductory chapter sets the scene, introducing the jigsaw model to the reader, providing a framework to explore each aspect of infant feeding care, described in subsequent chapters. Chapter 2 introduces the rationale for the development of positive and caring relationships between mothers and babies on the growth and functioning of the baby's brain. The importance of this and effective communication are thread throughout the book. Chapter 3 focuses on the anatomy and physiology of breastfeeding, and Chapter 4 goes on to highlight the value of skin-to-skin contact both on the relationship and closeness it enhances and the importance for the initiation and continuance of breastfeeding. Chapter 5 focuses on the skills required to support effective breastfeeding, and Chapter 6 explores the social context of feeding. In Chapter 7, the impact of contemporary birthing practices are discussed, followed by Chapter 8, which focuses on infant-feeding challenges related to the baby and how these might be resolved. In Chapter 9, the issues around formula feeding are addressed, including how responsive feeding can be achieved using this method. Then, in Chapter 10, the common maternal-related breastfeeding challenges are considered. Chapter 11 focuses on the premature infant and how breastfeeding can be supported for these vulnerable babies, and Chapter 12 concludes with an exploration of the valuable contributions made by the multi-agency team to the care of breastfeeding women. This book thoroughly prepares the reader to provide safe, evidence-based, woman-centred care for mothers as they learn to care for and feed their babies.

Huddersfield, Sheffield, Bournemouth 2017

Joyce Marshall
Helen Baston
Jenny Hall

Acknowledgements

In the process of writing, there are always people behind the scenes who support or add to the development of the book. We would specifically like to thank Mary Seager, formerly Senior Commissioning Editor at Elsevier, for her initial vision, support and prompting to turn the journal articles from *The Practising Midwife* into a readable volume. This project has now further developed with the insight and patience of Veronika Watkins and Alison Taylor. In addition, neither of us could have completed this second edition without the love, support and endless patience of our amazing families. To you, we owe our greatest gratitude.

CHAPTER 1

Introduction

This book is the fifth in the *Midwifery Essentials* series aimed at student midwives and those who support them in clinical practice. It focuses on infant feeding and relationship building between the mother and her new baby. It begins with the evidence regarding the effect of building positive, loving and caring relationships between mothers and babies and on growth and functioning of the baby's brain. It then considers the anatomy and physiology of breastfeeding and the skills that midwives use to support initiation and continuation of this vital process. Focus is then given to the social context of breastfeeding and addressing infant feeding challenges through multi-agency working. The UNICEF Baby Friendly Standards are thread throughout the book, enabling students to feel confident in the provision of evidence-based, family-centred care.

Scenarios are used throughout the book to facilitate learning and assist the reader to apply this knowledge to her own area of practice. The focus of contemporary maternity care is choice and continuity of care within a safe and effective service (Department of Health 2007; Maternity Review 2016). This book explores ways in which this aspiration can become a reality for women and their families.

The aim of this chapter is to:

+ Introduce the 'jigsaw model' for exploring effective midwifery practice.

The jigsaw model is used throughout the book with a view to helping midwives apply their knowledge in the provision of safe, effective compassionate care. It is used to explore the components of midwifery practice and apply them thoughtfully and intelligently to personalize care for each woman.

Midwifery care model

One of the purposes of this series is to consider the care of women and their babies from a holistic viewpoint. This means considering the care from a physical, emotional, psychological, spiritual, social and cultural

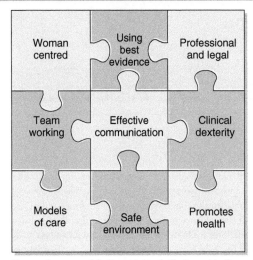

Woman centred	Using best evidence	Professional and legal
Team working	Effective communication	Clinical dexterity
Models of care	Safe environment	Promotes health

Fig. 1.1 Jigsaw model: dimensions of effective midwifery care.

context. To do this we have devised a jigsaw model of care that will encourage the reader to consider aspects of care while recognizing these aspects go to make up part of the whole person being cared for (Fig. 1.1).

This model will be used to reflect on the clinical scenarios described in the chapters. It shows the dimensions for effective maternity care, and each should be considered during the assessment, planning, implementation and evaluation of an aspect of care.

The pieces of the jigsaw clearly interlink with each other, and each is needed for the provision of safe, holistic care. When one is missing, the picture will be incomplete and care will not reach its potential. Each aspect of the model is described later in more detail. It is recommended that when an aspect of midwifery care is being evaluated, each piece of the jigsaw is addressed. Consider the questions pertaining to each piece of the jigsaw, and work through those that are relevant to the clinical situation you face.

Woman-centred care

The provision of woman-centred care was one of the central messages of the ground-breaking policy document *Changing Childbirth* (Department of Health 1993) which turned the focus of maternity care from meeting the needs of the professionals to listening and responding to the aspirations of women. This was further enforced in subsequent policy, including

Maternity Matters (Department of Health 2007) and ultimately in *Better Births* (Maternity Review 2016), a five-year-forward plan for maternity services. The central pillar of this vision is 'personalized care' underpinned by continuity of carer. When considering particular aspects of care, the questions that need to be addressed to ensure that the woman's care is woman-centred include:

+ Was the woman involved in the development of her care plan and its subsequent implementation?
+ Should her family or carers also be involved?
+ How can I ensure that she remains involved in further decisions about her care?
+ What are the implications of undertaking or not undertaking this procedure on this particular woman and baby?
+ Are there any factors that I need to consider that might influence the results of this procedure for this woman and its impact on her?
+ How does this procedure fit in with the woman's hopes and expectations?
+ Is now the most appropriate time to undertake this procedure?

Using best evidence

The Nursing and Midwifery Council Code of practice (NMC 2015:7) states you must deliver care 'on the basis of the best evidence and best practice … ensure any information or advice given is evidence-based'. There is a range of evidence to support the practice of midwifery (see Renfrew et al (2014) for a comprehensive summary of those practices that systematic reviews have shown to be effective). The decisions a midwife makes about her practice will be influenced by a range of factors. However, in the previous statement, care should be based as much as possible on the 'best evidence', whatever that may be. Questions that need to be addressed to ensure that the woman's care is evidence-based include:

+ What is already known about this aspect of care?
+ What is the research evidence available on this procedure?
+ Do local guidelines reflect best evidence?
+ Where can lay person's summaries of best practice be found?
+ Is there a National Institute for Health and Clinical Excellence (NICE) guideline about this issue?
+ What is the justification for the choices made about care?

Professional and legal

Midwives who practice in the United Kingdom must adhere to the rules and guidance of the Nursing and Midwifery Council (NMC). They are also required to comply with the law, rules and regulations of their employers.

Questions that need to be addressed to ensure that the woman's care fulfils statutory obligations include:

- Is this procedure expected to be an integral part of education prior to qualification?
- Which NMC proficiencies relate to this activity?
- How does The Code (NMC 2015) relate to this activity?
- Is there any other NMC guidance applicable to this activity?
- Are there any national or international guidelines for this activity?
- Are there any legal issues underpinning the use of this activity?
- What legislation applies to this context of working?

Team working

Midwives work as part of a team of professionals who each bring particular skills and perspectives to the care of women and their families. The Code (NMC 2015:8) requires registrants to 'work with colleagues to preserve the safety of those receiving care' and 'respect the skills, expertise and contributions of your colleagues, referring matters to them when appropriate'. The *midwives' rules and standards* (NMC 2012:15) provide further clarification and state that when a woman or baby's condition deviates from normal 'you must call such health or social care professionals as may reasonably be expected to have the necessary skills and experience to assist you in the provision of care'.

Questions that need to be addressed to ensure that the woman's care makes appropriate use of the multi-professional team include:

- Does this procedure fall within my role?
- Who else will need to be involved to interpret the results?
- Where should these results be recorded for all to see?
- Whom will I involve if the results are outside normal parameters?
- How can I facilitate effective team working with this woman?
- Will another person be required to assist with this procedure?
- When will they be available?

Effective communication

Central to any interaction between a woman and the midwife is effective communication. It is essential that the midwife is aware of the cues she is giving to the woman during the care she provides. Time is often pressured in midwifery, both in the community and hospital setting, but it is important to convey to the woman that she is the focus of your attention. Taking time to explain what you are going to do and why is crucial if she is going to trust that you are acting in her best interest. Effective communication is also essential between members of the multi-disciplinary team. Questions that need to be addressed to ensure that effective communication is achieved before, during and after this procedure include:

- What information needs to be given for the woman to choose whether this is the right form of care for her?
- Has she given consent?
- Is she clear as to what the care plan entails?
- In what ways could the information be given?
- What should be said during the administration of this care?
- What should be observed in the woman's behaviour during the activity?
- What should be communicated to the woman after the care has concluded?
- How and where should recording of the care and its impact be made?
- What communication tools are available to assist effective communication?

Clinical dexterity

Midwifery is a profession that requires the practitioner to have a range of knowledge and a repertoire of clinical skills. The midwife continues to learn new skills throughout her working life and is accountable for maintaining and developing her practice as new ways of working are introduced: 'Maintain the knowledge and skills you need for safe and effective practice' (NMC 2015:7).

Questions that need to be addressed to ensure that the woman's care is provided with clinical dexterity include:

- Can I practice this skill in other ways?
- How has my previous experience influenced how I approach this procedure today?
- How can I be sure I am carrying this out correctly?
- Am I using the most appropriate equipment for this task?
- Are there opportunities for practicing this skill elsewhere?

Models of care

Midwives work in many different settings and in a range of maternity care systems. For example, they may work independently providing holistic client-centred care, or they may work within a large tertiary centre providing care for women with complex health needs. The models of care can be influential in determining the care that a woman may receive, from whom and when. Midwives need to consider the most appropriate ways that care can be delivered so that they can influence future development in the best interests of women and their families.

Questions that need to be addressed to ensure that the impact of the way that care is provided is acknowledged include:

+ How is the maternity service organized?
+ Which professional groups are involved in the provision of this service?
+ How is this procedure influenced by the model of care provided?
+ How does this model of care impact on the carers?
+ How does this model of care impact on the woman and her family?

Safe environment

The code states that 'you must act without delay if you believe that there is a risk to patient safety or public protection' (NMC 2015:12). The midwife must ensure that the care she gives does not compromise the safety of women and their families. She must therefore create and maintain a safe working environment at all times, wherever she practices. Questions that need to be addressed to ensure that the woman's care is provided in a safe environment include:

+ Are there facilities to ensure that her privacy and dignity are maintained?
+ Is there somewhere to wash hands?
+ Is there an appropriate place to dispose of waste?
+ Is the equipment appropriately maintained and free from contamination?
+ Is the space adequate to allow ease of movement around the woman without invading her personal space?
+ What are the risks involved in this procedure and how have they been addressed?
+ Are there any risks to the person undertaking the procedure?
+ Is this environment safe for others who might come into the room?

Promotes health

Providing care for women and their families presents a unique opportunity to influence the health and wellbeing of the public. Midwives must capitalize on their contacts with women to help them achieve a healthy pregnancy and birth and promote lifestyle choices that will benefit women, babies and families in the future. Questions that need to be addressed to ensure that the woman's care promotes health include:

+ Is this procedure going to help her or harm her or her baby in any way?
+ What are the opportunities to use this procedure to educate her and her family on healthy behaviour?
+ What resources can women and families access to help them make healthy lifestyle choices?

+ How can I motivate a woman without jeopardizing my relationship with her?

The book begins with a chapter focusing on relationship building. As the jigsaw model shows, effective communication is central to the provision of woman-centred midwifery care. The following chapters then use the jigsaw model to explore scenarios from practice. Thus the reader is provided with a structure with which to reflect on her care and that of the multi-professional team in which she works. Each chapter includes a range of activities designed to enable the midwife to contextualize the information within her own practice, applying her continually developing knowledge to her own circumstances. The chapters are written so that they can be accessed without the previous ones having been read, although we hope you will find the whole book relevant and thought provoking. Enjoy!

References

Department of Health, 1993. Changing Childbirth: Report of the Expert maternity Group Pt. II; Report of the Expert Maternity Group Pt. I. Department of Health, London.

Department of Health, 2007. Maternity Matters: Choice, access and continuity of care in a safe service. Available at: http://webarchive.nationalarchives.gov.uk/20130107105354/http://www.dh.gov.uk/prod_consum_dh/groups/dh_digitalassets/@dh/@en/documents/digitalasset/dh_074199.pdf.

Maternity Review, 2016. Better Births. Improving outcomes of maternity services in England, a five year forward view for maternity care. Available at: https://www.england.nhs.uk/wp-content/uploads/2016/02/national-maternity-review-report.pdf.

Nursing and Midwifery Council, 2012. Midwives rules and standards. https://www.nmc.org.uk/globalassets/sitedocuments/standards/nmc-midwives-rules-and-standards.pdf.

Nursing and Midwifery Council, 2015. The code: Professional standards of practice and behaviour for nurses and midwives. Available at: https://www.nmc.org.uk/globalassets/sitedocuments/nmc-publications/nmc-code.pdf.

Renfrew, M., Mcfadden, A., Bastos, H., et al., 2014. Midwifery and quality care: Findings from a new evidence-informed framework for maternal and newborn care. Lancet 384 (9948), 1129–1145.

Relationship building between mother and baby

TRIGGER SCENARIO

Maria is 25 weeks' pregnant, and she is at a clinic in the local health centre talking to her community midwife, Sarah. They are chatting about how Maria thinks about her baby. As she rubs her baby bump, Maria tells Sarah with a laugh that she calls the baby 'Tiddlywinks' and that she talks to her 'all the time'. She says 'we found out at the scan that she is a girl, and I bet she will be energetic as she moves a lot when I listen to the radio in the morning'.

Introduction

The environment and events that occur during pregnancy, childbirth and early after birth have potential to affect the health and wellbeing of the baby not just at that time but throughout their life span (Moore et al 2012). There is also increasing evidence that the health and wellbeing of future generations may be 'programmed' by events at these critical times (Barker 2012). Therefore support provided by midwives and other health professionals to help mothers maintain good physical and emotional health during pregnancy and develop a nurturing and caring environment for their baby after birth is crucial.

Having a new baby in the family is often a joyous occasion, but there is no doubt that it is a time of great social and psychological change that many women find challenging. It is important therefore that care provided is holistic, focusing not only on physical care but also addressing women's emotional and psychological needs in the context of their family situation as they make the transition to motherhood (Royal College of Midwives (RCM) 2012). This is in line with the World Health Organization (1948) definition of health as:

> 'a state of complete physical, mental and social wellbeing and not merely the absence of disease or infirmity'.

Research on how babies develop emotional and behavioural wellbeing within the relationship with their caregivers, combined with advances in neuroscience and epigenetics, provides strong evidence of the importance of this relationship to future health and wellbeing. Infant feeding inevitably occurs within this relationship between a mother and her baby and can strengthen the relationship or impact negatively on it if the mother does not get helpful support when she needs it.

UNICEF Baby Friendly Maternity standards

The following are the maternity standards that are most relevant to this chapter:

- Support pregnant women to recognize the importance of breastfeeding and early relationships for the health and wellbeing of their baby
- Support parents to have a close and loving relationship with their baby

---

UNICEF Baby Friendly UK University learning outcomes

The following are the learning outcomes that are achieved within this chapter. By the end of their midwifery education programme, students will:

- Develop an understanding of the importance of secure mother-infant attachment and the impact this has on their health and emotional wellbeing
- Be able to apply their knowledge of attachment theory to promote and encourage close and loving relationships between mothers and babies
- Have the knowledge and skills to access the evidence that underpins infant feeding practice
- Be able to apply their knowledge of effective communication to initiate sensitive, mother-centred conversations with pregnant women and new mothers

---

Why relationships matter to babies' health and wellbeing

How environment affects genes: epigenetics

When the sequencing of the human genome was completed in 2003, it became apparent that genetic make-up alone could not explain the massive variation in human characteristics and conditions, and this increased interest in the study of epigenetics (Rivera & Bennett 2010). At the simplest level, epigenetics is the science of how genes are expressed; that is which ones are switched on or off. The epigenome is the link between genetics and the environment. It is a complex marking of the DNA which is sensitive to and modified by the environment that ultimately can control factors such as development and disease susceptibility.

Epigenetic processes are dynamic, not fixed, although some do persist for long periods of time and can be inherited. Factors such as a healthy diet and positive social interactions can encourage beneficial epigenetic markers and gene expression. However, traumatic experiences in early life and chronic stress can encourage less beneficial epigenetic markers (Suderman et al 2014) and therefore impact negatively on the child's development and susceptibility to chronic disease in adulthood.

Activity

Revise your knowledge of basic genetics and then search the Internet for either an article or a video clip of how epigenetics works and why it is important. Ensure you have a basic understanding of processes such as DNA methylation, histone modification, the role of protein complexes and micros RNA. This link is a helpful one: https://www.youtube.com/watch?v=9DAcJSAM_BA.

Development of a baby's brain and the neuroscience of caring

In the early weeks of pregnancy, there is rapid development of the fetal brain, and at 20 weeks' gestation, all major anatomical parts of the brain and the DNA template are in place. Further development after this is affected by conditions experienced by the developing fetus (Bergman 2013). Neurons form in the brain until 28 weeks; once formed, they migrate to other parts of the brain and make connections to sensory organs. The sensitive nature of these cells means that various sensations cause them to release an action potential or 'fire' which encourages further cell development. Repeated firing leads to stabilization of synapses, and those that are not stabilized are eliminated. It is the combination of these two processes that establishes neural pathways in the baby's brain. Some parts of the brain are 'hardwired' by birth, such as the brain stem which controls physical functions like breathing and heart rate, but other parts of the brain, such as the limbic system which control moods and emotions, continue to develop until the child is aged 3 years. During this time, family relationships and the caring or otherwise within the child's environment can have significant impact on their future health and wellbeing.

There are critical periods of time when a child's brain is susceptible to adverse events and around the time of birth is one of these. At this time, skin-to-skin contact between mother and baby provides stimuli for the infant such as warmth, smell and movement. This is the way that the baby learns what is normal and 'sets the platform for future emotional and social intelligence' (Bergman 2013:48). Quality sensory experiences between mother and baby during the first 8 weeks of the baby's life set pathways in the brain that affect emotional health and behaviour in the future.

Activity

Go to http://www.your-baby.org.uk/ and consider how this website promoting emotional wellbeing before and after birth might help women to develop relationships with their baby.

Supporting women to build a relationship with their baby before birth

Encouraging women to start to build a relationship with their baby before the baby is born can provide a good foundation (Entwistle 2013). This is a key part of the role of the midwife and can happen during routine antenatal contacts and/or during antenatal education sessions. Antenatal education sessions available to women in different areas vary greatly and are not always provided by midwives or considered to be a priority by trusts. A review of antenatal education concluded that parenting begins before the baby is born and that antenatal education should include preparation for the transition to parenthood (Barlow et al 2009). This is now becoming more common and is supported by NICE antenatal care guidelines that state 'pregnant women should be offered opportunities to attend participant-led antenatal classes' (NICE 2008).

Women are particularly receptive to information during pregnancy and usually want to do what is best for their baby. It is a time when women may be more likely to ask for help if they are struggling with, for example, partner abuse (Cuthbert et al 2011). Conversations during pregnancy should be focused on parents' individual hopes and needs, should take into account their broader social context and should aim to build their confidence and self-efficacy. Discussions about infant feeding may be part of this.

Many factors can impact on a woman's ability to start to relate to her baby during pregnancy. Some examples include: whether the pregnancy was planned or not, drug and alcohol use, mental health issues and domestic abuse (Cuthbert et al 2011). A woman's level of engagement with her baby can be assessed by talking to her about her unborn baby and understanding how she visualizes and imagines her baby (RCM 2012).

Activity

Ask the next few pregnant women you meet how they think about and imagine their babies. Compare these and consider what family traditions, relationships and influences may have contributed to these images. What might you suggest to encourage mothers to interact with their baby?

The early hours after birth

The intense emotional feelings experienced by most mothers towards their baby after birth is the continuation of the relationship that started during pregnancy and is referred to as *bonding*. Many mothers feel these emotions soon after birth, but for some this can take longer, particularly if the birth has not lived up to the mothers' expectations or has been traumatic (RCM 2012). If mothers do not feel this connection with their baby, it can be a source of worry for them. When women have close bodily contact with their baby, this releases oxytocin which can help to encourage her to feel this connection. Spending time in skin-to-skin contact with her baby means she is more likely to interact with her baby demonstrating behaviours such as stroking and talking to her baby. Skin-to-skin contact also helps the baby make the transition to extra-uterine life and reduces stress in the baby.

Activity

One-to-one care for women in labour can impact positively on their ability to build a relationship with their baby (Entwistle 2013). Consider how you might encourage a woman to make connections with her baby when you are caring for her in labour.

Supporting relationship building between mother and baby in the postnatal period

To support women to develop a positive relationship with their baby, it is important to understand the concepts of bonding and attachment and to consider circumstances that might impact on these.

Bonding and attachment

There is not a single clear definition of bonding, and it is often conflated and confused with the concept of attachment. However, most authors agree that bonding is the one-way intense emotional tie felt by a mother for her infant (Bicking Kinsey & Hupcey 2013). Babies can interact socially from the moment they are born. They make eye contact, follow movement with their eyes and appear to listen. Most mothers feel a strong need to respond when their baby cries.

The seminal work on bonding by Klaus and Kennell (1976) suggested the presence of a critical period early after birth when bonding occurs. In the 1970s this may have been helpful, discouraging the common practice of separating mothers and babies after birth. However, the idea of a critical period can also be a source of worry for mothers who are separated from their baby by necessity, for example, if the baby requires special care. More recently it has been suggested that although this close contact immediately after birth is desirable, bonding between mother and baby can occur over a longer period of time (Crouch & Manderson 1995; Kennell & McGrath 2005).

Attachment is different to bonding in that it refers to the infant rather than the mother. A definition of attachment is the formation of a strong emotional relationship of the baby or infant with a primary caregiver. The concept was first studied in the 1950s by Bowlby who suggested that a strong attachment provides an infant with a foundation and security from which to explore the world. Ainsworth developed some of Bowlby's ideas further and through observational research of 'the strange situation' identified types of attachment behaviours. These were further developed by Main, a student of Ainsworth, and are summarized in Table 2.1.

A secure attachment relationship develops over time and in relation to the responses of the primary caregiver (usually the mother). When a mother is sensitive to her infant's needs and responds to them, the infant develops trust and confidence. Securely attached infants seek attention from their mothers, are distressed when their mothers leave but are consoled on her return. The majority of infants (around 65%–70%) display this behaviour. Insecure-avoidant infants are not as affected by the mother's departure and, upon her return, will not approach her but may avoid her. Insecure-resistant infants are distressed when the mother leaves and, upon

Table 2.1: **Types of attachment**

Quality of caregiving	Strategy to deal with distress	Type of attachment
Sensitive, loving	Organized	Secure
Insensitive, rejecting	Organized	Insecure-avoidant
Insensitive, inconsistent	Organized	Insecure-resistant
Atypical	Disorganized	Insecure-disorganized

Adapted from (Benoit 2004).

her return, are torn between the need for closeness and resisting comfort. A small minority of infants display disorganized behaviour, which is an unpredictable pattern of behaviour on the mother's return.

This is important because children with insecure or disorganized attachment have been shown to be more affected by stressful situations and find it more difficult to control negative emotions in later life. They are also more likely to have lower self-esteem and confidence, and to find it more difficult to form peer relationships (Benoit 2004).

The transition to parenthood is not always easy. For example, a new baby can change and sometime put strain on parental relationships. Factors such as drug or alcohol misuse, postnatal depression and domestic abuse may mean that it is more difficult for an infant to build an attachment relationship with their parents (RCM 2012). For women experiencing challenges, their babies may benefit most from support during pregnancy, childbirth and the early postnatal period. Facilitating the development of relationships that are as strong and loving as possible can go some way to reducing the effects of adversity by creating resilience in the child (Kiernan & Mensah 2011).

REFLECTION ON THE TRIGGER SCENARIO

Look back at the trigger scenario.

> Maria is 25 weeks' pregnant, and she is at a clinic in the local health centre talking to her community midwife, Sarah. They are chatting about how Maria thinks about her baby. As she rubs her baby bump, Maria tells Sarah with a laugh that she calls the baby 'Tiddlywinks' and that she talks to her 'all the time'. She says 'we found out at the scan that she is a girl, and I bet she will be energetic as she moves a lot when I listen to the radio in the morning'.

Sarah is visiting Maria at home after the birth of her baby, Lucy. Sarah notices that Maria appears to be rather tearful and asks 'how are things going?' Maria has just finished breastfeeding and is cuddling Lucy, gazing down at her as she sleeps peacefully. Maria appears worried and explains to Sarah that she doesn't feel she is bonding with Lucy as she thought she would.

This scenario highlights one mother's concern about her emotions towards her baby. Often, mothers create a picture of how they will feel and the bond they will have with their baby. This can be based on media representations and other people's ideas and expectations. If a mother's feelings do not match with her expectations, this may be a source of worry impacting on her confidence in the early days with a new baby. However, if Sarah is able to spend time listening to Maria and reassuring her that her instinctive nurturing behaviour is helping Lucy's development, she may be able to allay Maria's anxiety and help to build her confidence.

Now that you are familiar with important aspects of relationship building between a mother and her baby, you should have insight into how the scenario relates to the evidence. The jigsaw model will now be used to explore the trigger scenario in more depth.

Effective communication

It is essential that midwives communicate effectively with women about building a relationship with their baby during antenatal appointments and after the birth of the baby. Sarah provided Maria with these opportunities to discuss her feelings towards her baby and to express any concerns. Involving partners in such discussions may also be helpful. Questions that arise from the scenario might include: Sarah had developed a relationship with Maria before the birth of her baby – how might this have helped communication during postnatal visits? What non-verbal communication might Sarah have used when she noticed that Maria was upset? What questions could the midwife ask if a woman does not spontaneously discuss her feeling towards her baby? What signs might the midwife notice if a mother is not bonding well with her baby?

Woman-centred care

Midwives should provide sensitive, individualized care for women, and this will involve recognizing when women might need more opportunity to discuss their feelings during the transition to motherhood. Women develop relationships with their baby in different ways and within varied contexts. Questions that arise from the scenario might include: Might it have been helpful to Maria to discuss her birth experience if this was not in line with her expectations? If Maria had experienced depression during the antenatal period, is this likely to impact on her ability to develop a relationship with her baby? Maria has chosen to breastfeed, so how might this help or hinder her developing relationship with her baby?

Using best evidence

There is considerable evidence about the importance of a nurturing relationship between mother and baby and that this should begin during pregnancy and develop throughout the early years. Questions that can be addressed to ensure a woman's care is evidence-based include: What resources can the midwife provide for women about developing a relationship with their baby? Is there an evidence-based mobile phone application that might help some women to understand the developmental stage of their baby during pregnancy? How will Sarah use National Guidelines to enable her to provide the most appropriate care for Maria?

Professional and legal issues

Midwives must practice within a professional and legal framework to maintain high standards of care. The professional standards of practice outlined in The Code (NMC 2015) require midwives to practice in line with the best available evidence and to act in the best interests of people at all times. In this scenario, questions that need to be addressed to ensure that care fulfils statutory obligations include: How will the midwife ensure she makes adequate time within the context of busy antenatal and postnatal care to enable meaningful conversations with women? What local and national guidelines might relate to Maria's and Lucy's care? How would the midwife document care provided for Maria and Lucy?

Team working

In addition to community midwifery services, most women in the UK receive ongoing care from a health visitor usually until their child is 5 years old. Questions that might arise from this scenario include: How does the health visitor receive notification that the midwife is no longer visiting? Will the health visitor have already met Maria? If so, when will this have been? If Maria has extra needs, who else might be involved in her care? Are there any social groups for new parents in your area that women like Maria might find helpful?

Clinical dexterity

The midwife supporting a woman to build a positive relationship with her baby will need to understand the importance of this and the underpinning evidence of the effect on the baby's development and future wellbeing. The most important skill in this scenario will be sensitive communication that will enable Maria to discuss her feelings and any concerns she may have. Questions that arise from the scenario might include: What do women expect from the midwife providing antenatal and postnatal care? How can you ensure you listen as well as provide information? How might Sarah increase Maria's knowledge and build her confidence? How might sensitive infant feeding support contribute to Maria's developing relationship with Lucy?

Models of care

It is not clear from the scenario what model of care Maria had received when giving birth to Lucy, but she had developed an ongoing relationship with Sarah during pregnancy and this continued during the postnatal period. It is possible that Sarah was present during birth, but this is not likely unless team midwifery is the model of care available to Maria. Questions that arise from the scenario might include: How might the model of care Maria received influence her developing relationship with Lucy? What models of care are available to women in your area of practice? Would continuity of care be beneficial to Maria? If so, why might this be helpful? If there is not continuity of care, do the maternity records provide sufficient detail to enable other midwives to follow Maria's progress?

Safe environment

Sarah has a responsibility to ensure that Maria and Lucy and other women in her care are in an environment that is as safe as possible. Questions that arise from the scenario might include: Is Maria in a safe environment at home or are there reasons why she or Lucy may be at risk? When a woman feels more relaxed, she is more likely to spontaneously interact with her baby; what can Sarah do to encourage Maria to feel more relaxed when visiting her at home in the postnatal period? How might Sarah enable Maria to express any concerns she may have?

Promotes health

The midwife has a key role to play in promoting the health and wellbeing of the woman and her baby. Helping each woman to adapt to motherhood and to build a nurturing relationship with her baby will potentially have long-lasting positive effects on the baby's emotional and behavioural health. Questions that might arise from the scenario include: Are there ways that Sarah could further promote Maria's emotional health? Would it be beneficial to involve Maria's partner? If so, how might she do this? Are there resources Sarah could use to help?

Further scenarios

The following scenarios enable you to consider how specific situations influence the care the midwife provides. Use the jigsaw model to explore the issues raised in the scenario.

Libby had her baby, James, 5 days ago. She explains to Veronica, the community midwife who is visiting her at home, that James is breastfeeding often. Libby says, 'I feel like he is using me as a dummy'.

Practice point

It is common to hear breastfeeding women make comments like this, and it is important for the midwife to listen carefully and build on Libby's existing knowledge to convey the message that comfort is as important as nutrition to a baby's health and wellbeing.

Further points specific to Scenario 1 include:
1. If you were the midwife caring for Libby and James, what would you say to enable you to maximize their health and wellbeing in line with The Code (NMC 2015)?
2. How might you start a conversation to explore Libby's feelings towards James?
3. What kinds of things might you suggest that Libby could do enhance her relationship with James?
4. What evidence might you draw upon to support your discussion?
5. How might you involve Libby's partner?

Lindsey has chosen to bottle feed her baby girl, Freya, who was born earlier this morning. Helen is the midwife caring for Lindsey today on the postnatal ward. Freya is just starting to stir, and Lindsey has asked Helen what she should do and asks 'does Freya need a feed?'

Practice point

It is arguably even more important to encourage women who have chosen to bottle feed to build a relationship with their baby as they are perhaps less likely to be the person that feeds their baby every time. It is important to limit the number of different people who bottle feed a baby as this does not enhance bonding and attachment between mother and baby (UNICEF Baby Friendly Initiative UK 2014).

Further points specific to Scenario 2 include:
1. What hormone is likely to be reduced if Lindsey does not keep Freya near her and bottle feed her herself?
2. How would you encourage Lindsey to build a positive relationship with Freya?

3. Lindsey appears to be recognizing Freya's feeding cues; how might you build on this to encourage responsive feeding?
4. What would you explain to Lindsey to ensure she bottle feeds Freya safely?
5. What resources might you provide for Lindsey?

Conclusion

The importance of environmental conditions for babies, such as adequate nutrition for mothers during pregnancy and building a positive and nurturing relationship with parents, can be considered to be the cornerstone to improving the health of the population in the future. Various fields of science have provided evidence of the potential to improve children's ability to cope with stress, enhance their brain development and reduce the risk of chronic diseases in adulthood. Therefore midwives have a key role to play by providing education and support to families in a balanced and sensitive way that does not induce feelings of pressure or guilt but that enhances emotional wellbeing.

Resources

Entwistle, F.M. 2013) The evidence and rationale for the UNICEF UK Baby Friendly Initiative standards. UNICEF UK. Available at: http://www.unicef.org.uk/Documents/Baby_Friendly/Research/baby_friendly_evidence_rationale.pdf.

NICE 2010. Pregnancy and complex social factors: a model for service provision for pregnant women with complex social factors. NICE Clinical Guideline 110. National Collaborating Centre for Women's and Children's Health.

NICE 2014. Antenatal and postnatal mental health: clinical management and service guidance. NICE Clinical Guideline 192. National Collaborating Centre for Women's and Children's Health.

NICE 2016. Antenatal care for uncomplicated pregnancies. NICE Clinical Guideline 62. National Collaborating Centre for Women's and Children's Health.

UNICEF Baby Friendly Initiative. Building a Happy Baby leaflet. Available at: http://www.unicef.org.uk/BabyFriendly/Resources/Resources-for-parents/Building-a-happy-baby/.

UNICEF Baby Friendly Initiative. Importance of relationship building video. Available at: http://www.unicef.org.uk/BabyFriendly/Resources/Resources-for-parents/Building-a-happy-baby/.

References

Barker, D.J.P., 2012. Developmental origins of chronic disease. Public Health 126, 185–189.

Barlow, J., Coe, C., Redshaw, M., Underdown, A., 2009. Birth and beyond: Stakeholder perceptions of current antenatal education provision in England. Warwick Infant and Family Wellbeing Unit, University of Warwick, National Perinatal Epidemiology Unit, Oxford.

Benoit, D., 2004. Infant-parent attachment: Definition, types, antecedents, measurement and outcome. Paediatr. Child Health 9, 541–545.

Bergman, N., 2013. Breastfeeding and perinatal neuroscience. In: Watson Genna, C. (Ed.), Supporting sucking skills in breastfeeding infants, 2nd ed. Jones and Bartlett, Burlington.

Bicking Kinsey, C., Hupcey, J.E., 2013. State of the science of maternal-infant bonding: a principle-based concept analysis. Midwifery 29, doi:10.1016/j.midw.2012.1012.1019.

Crouch, M., Manderson, L., 1995. The social life of bonding theory. Soc. Sci. Med. 41, 837–844.

Cuthbert, C., Rayns, G., Stanley, K., 2011. All babies count: Prevention and protection for vulnerable babies. NSPCC. Available at: https://http://www.nspcc.org.uk/globalassets/documents/research-reports/all-babies-count-prevention-protection-vulnerable-babies-report.pdf.

Entwistle, F.M., 2013. The evidence and rationale for the UNICEF UK Baby Friendly Initiative standards. UNICEF UK.

Kennell, J., McGrath, S., 2005. Starting the process of mother–infant bonding. Acta Paediatr. 94, 775–777.

Kiernan, K.E., Mensah, F.K., 2011. Poverty, family resources and children's early educational attainment: The mediating role of parenting. Br. Educ. Res. J. 37, 317–336.

Klaus, M.H., Kennell, J.H., 1976. Maternal-Infant Bonding. The C.V Mosby Company, St. Louis.

Moore, E.R., Anderson, G.C., Bergman, N., Dowswell, T., 2012. Early skin-to-skin contact for mothers and their healthy newborn infants. Cochrane Database Syst. Rev. (5), Art. No.: CD003519, doi:10.1002/14651858.CD003519.pub3.

NICE, 2008. Antenatal care for uncomplicated pregnancies. NICE Clinical Guideline 62. National Collaborating Centre for Women's and Children's Health.

NMC, 2015. The code: professional standards of practice and behaviour for nurses and midwives. Nursing and Midwifery Council, London. Available at: https://http://www.nmc.org.uk/globalassets/sitedocuments/nmc-publications/nmc-code.pdf.

RCM, 2012. Maternal emotional wellbeing and infant development: A good practice guide for midwives.

Rivera, R.M., Bennett, L.B., 2010. Epigenetics in humans: an overview. Curr. Opin. Endocrinol. Diabetes Obes. 17, 493–499.

Suderman, M., Borghol, N., Pappas, J.J., et al., 2014. Childhood abuse is associated with methylation of multiple loci in adult DNA. BMC Med. Genomics 7, 1755–8794.

UNICEF Baby Friendly Initiative UK, 2014. The UNICEF UK Baby Friendly Initiative Train the Trainer. UNICEF Baby Friendly Initiative UK, London.

World Health Organization, 1948. Preamble to the Constitution of the World Health Organization as adopted by the International Health Conference, New York, 19 June - 22 July 1946; signed on 22 July 1946 by the representatives of 61 States (Official Records of the World Health Organization, no. 2, p. 100) and entered into force on 7 April 1948. Available at: http://www.who.int/governance/eb/who_constitution_en.pdf.

CHAPTER 3

Anatomy and physiology

TRIGGER SCENARIO

Harry is a few hours old and is beginning to stir in his cot. He opens his eyes, lifts his head slightly and yawns. Emma, his mother, watches him sleepily from her bed wondering if he is ready for another breastfeed. Slowly, feeling rather sore, she eases herself out of bed and lifts him out of the cot. Murmuring softly to him, she settles into the chair beside the bed and holds him close to her; as she touches his cheek, he turns his head towards her and opens his mouth. 'You're hungry, aren't you Harry,' she says and prepares to breastfeed him.

Introduction

For midwives to support women who have chosen to breastfeed effectively, it is essential that they provide women with good up-to-date, evidence-based information. In 2010 in the UK, around 81% of women started to breastfeed their babies, but by 6 weeks only around 23% of women were still breastfeeding (Health and Social Care Information Centre 2012). A range of cultural, psychosocial and practical factors may influence women's decisions at this time, but it is likely that if women receive clear and useful information and emotional support as they start to breastfeed, they will build a good relationship with their baby and enjoy breastfeeding. This chapter outlines the basic knowledge of anatomy and physiology required by midwives to underpin the information and support they provide for breastfeeding women. This includes an understanding of the external and internal anatomy of the breast, the mechanism of suckling, the innate infant reflexes that enable a newborn to breastfeed instinctively and the physiology of lactation.

UNICEF Baby Friendly Maternity standards

The following are the maternity standards that are most relevant to this chapter:
- Enable mothers to get breastfeeding off to a good start
- Support mothers to make informed decisions regarding the introduction of food or fluids other than breast milk

---

Anatomy of the breast

The breast is made up of glandular and adipose tissue supported by Cooper's ligaments (a framework of fibrous connective tissue) and lies over the pectoral muscles of the chest wall. Externally, the nipple is in the centre of the areola, which is a darker pigmented area. There is variation in the size and shape of women's nipples and the size and colour of the areola. Within the areola are sebaceous glands called *Montgomery's tubercles*. These secrete an oily substance that lubricates the nipple, protects against infection and is believed to provide a scent that guides a newborn infant to the nipple (Wambach & Riordan 2015). During pregnancy, the breasts increase in size, the areola darkens in colour and Mongomery's tubercles become bigger (Geddes 2007a).

The glandular tissue within the lactating breast is made up of alveoli. Each of these is a cluster of acini (milk-producing gland) cells surrounded by myoepithelial (muscle) cells that eject milk into the ducts. Between 10 and 100 alveoli are grouped into lobes that are entwined and interconnected (Geddes 2007b). Milk is continuously secreted into the alveoli where it is stored until the muscle cells contract to eject the milk into the ducts. These join together, rather like the branches of a tree, to become single ducts that pass through and open at the end of the nipple.

The internal anatomy of the breast has relatively recently been investigated using high resolution ultrasound, and this has led to revised descriptions of breast anatomy. Research by Ramsey et al (2005) showed

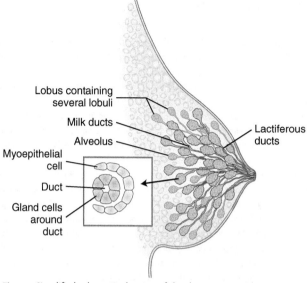

Lobus containing
several lobuli

Milk ducts

Alveolus

Myoepithelial
cell

Duct

Gland cells
around
duct

Lactiferous
ducts

Fig. 3.1 Simplified schematic drawing of the duct system with cross-section of myoepithethelial cells around the duct. Myoepithelial cells contract to eject milk.

that there are between 4 and 18 ducts at the nipple (mean of 9) and that these ducts branch close to the nipple (Fig. 3.1). Although they widen at multiple branch points, there are no sinuses as previously described. Lactiferous ducts are small, superficial, intertwined and easily compressed. Their function is now thought to be transport rather than storage (Geddes 2007b). It is important that mothers understand that breasts do not store large quantities of milk (i.e. are not containers of milk) but rather that breast milk is produced constantly in small amounts.

Activity

What aspects of the anatomy of the breast are important for women to know to enable them to understand the flexible nature of breastfeeding? Breasts vary greatly in size and shape. Do women with larger breasts produce more breast milk? What kind of tissue is there more of in a larger breast?

How a baby breastfeeds (mechanism of suckling/reflexes)

It is important to consider how a baby breastfeeds in relation to the anatomy of the breast especially in the light of the recent knowledge that lactiferous sinuses do not exist. It is generally believed that breast milk is removed by peristaltic action of the infant's tongue on the roof of the mouth; however, recent ultrasound studies have demonstrated that milk flows into the infant's mouth when a vacuum is created by lowering of the infant's tongue (Geddes 2007b), and this vacuum is likely to be an important aspect of milk removal. This may be important in clinical practice to enable diagnosis and management of infants with sucking abnormalities.

The newborn's mouth is well designed for suckling; the normal resting position of the tongue is with the tip over the bottom lip where it can easily make contact with the breast (Genna & Sandora 2013). The lips are flexible and, when breastfeeding, the lower lip is usually rolled outward, but if the upper lip is also turned out, this can be a sign of poor attachment. Newborns have good airway protection in that the epiglottis and soft palate touch at rest; this and the short upper airway reduce the risk of aspiration. Infants are born with three reflexes that are important to enable them to breastfeed: 1. The rooting reflex – when something touches the cheek the infant turns the head, opens the mouth and brings the tongue down and forward; 2. The sucking reflex – when something touches the infant's palate, the infant sucks to draw it into the mouth and 3. The swallowing reflex – when the mouth fills with milk, the infant raises the jaw to swallow (UNICEF Baby Friendly Initiative UK 2014). These later two reflexes are coordinated for a baby to feed.

Activity

Watch the video clip of a peer supporter helping a breastfeeding woman to position and attach her baby at https://www.unicef.org.uk/babyfriendly/baby-friendly-resources/video/positioning-and-attachment/ and the short clip on the biological nurturing website on laid-back breastfeeding at http://www.biologicalnurturing.com/video/bn3clip.html. Consider how the reflexes the baby is born with help in each of these situations.

Physiology of lactation

Prolactin

Prolactin is the hormone responsible for production of breast milk. During pregnancy, levels of prolactin increase steadily but are inhibited by high levels of progesterone. Once the placenta has been expelled, levels become higher and this, combined with suckling, initiates lactation. Prolactin is secreted by the anterior pituitary gland into the blood stream in response to suckling and nipple stimulation and acts on receptor sites on the walls of the acini cells to synthesize milk. It is secreted during breastfeeding and levels peak about 40 to 45 minutes after a feed, acting on the acini cells in both breasts to produce milk for the next feed. Prolactin levels are highest at night as they follow a circadian rhythm (Wambach & Riordan 2015). There is a theory that the initial release of prolactin after birth primes and stimulates prolactin receptor sites in the acini cells and that frequent milk removal in the early days primes more receptor sites leading to improved milk production (Pollard 2012).

Activity

How do you think a retained segment of placenta might affect breastfeeding? What suggestions might you offer a woman who desperately wants to breastfeed but is very tired following the birth of her baby? Consider routines of care in your unit both around birth and postnatally, what more could be done to ensure women have early opportunity to breastfeed after birth and continuing support to ensure feeding gets off to a good start?

Oxytocin

Oxytocin is responsible for milk ejection – the 'let-down' reflex. It is released from the posterior pituitary gland and acts on the myoepithelial cells that surround the alveoli to move milk from the alveoli into the ducts. Shortening of the ducts increases pressure helping to eject milk and duct diameter increases. Levels of oxytocin in the blood rise within 1 minute of stimulation, and this is essential for breastfeeding as only small volumes of milk (1–10 ml) can be removed by the infant before milk ejection (Geddes 2007b). In the first few days after birth the let-down reflex is stimulated by the infant suckling and by the mother seeing, touching, hearing and smelling her baby but can (usually in the short term) be inhibited by anxiety and stress. Some women sense the let-down reflex as a sensation within their breast whereas others do not. As breastfeeding continues the let-down reflex can occur in response to other stimuli such as hearing another child crying or thinking about feeding. As well as stimulating milk ejection, oxytocin also dilates blood vessels on the chest meaning that mothers transfer warmth to their baby. Oxytocin contributes to increased maternal interaction and bonding, enhances the mother's sense of wellbeing and may even be health-promoting (Uvnas-Moberg & Petersson 2005).

> **Activity**
>
> Speak to several women who have or are breastfeeding and ask them what sensations (if any) they experience as the milk starts to flow. Do women experience this during a feed as well as at the beginning? Access your trust breastfeeding policy and look for recommendations that affect breastfeeding hormones. How might you encourage a mother who is anxious to relax so that oxytocin is released and the let-down reflex occurs?

Feedback inhibitor of lactation

Feedback inhibitor of lactation (FIL) is whey protein that is produced by acini cells and inhibits milk production at the local level (i.e. in each breast independently). As the alveoli distend with milk, the concentration of FIL increases and it is this rather than pressure that controls the amount of milk produced. When milk is removed concentrations of FIL drop and milk is synthesized once more (Pollard 2012).

> **Activity**
>
> If a woman's breasts are very full and the baby is unable to latch onto the breast to feed, what would you suggest to her to ensure a continuing good milk supply and to reduce the effect of FIL? What would happen if a woman consistently breastfed from one breast only and did not touch the other?

REFLECTION ON THE TRIGGER SCENARIO

Look back at the trigger scenario.

> *Harry is a few hours old and is beginning to stir in his cot. He opens his eyes, lifts his head slightly and yawns. Emma, his mother, watches him sleepily from her bed wondering if he is ready for another breastfeed. Slowly, feeling rather sore, she eases herself out of bed and lifts him out of the cot. Murmuring softly to him, she settles into the chair beside the bed and holds him close to her; as she touches his cheek, he turns his head towards her and opens his mouth. 'You're hungry, aren't you Harry,' she says and prepares to breastfeed him.*

Harry is displaying several signs of a baby who is ready to breastfeed. Emma responds to these cues and confidently starts to breastfeed even though she is tired from giving birth. Early recognition of feeding cues is important as breastfeeding is often easier at this time. Once a baby is crying, a valuable opportunity has been missed. What information about feeding might Emma have been given or experienced? Who might have provided this information and when? Might she have seen breastfeeding mothers at a local Baby Bistro or Children's Centre? What support might Harry and Emma require at this time? How would early support for breastfeeding mothers be provided in your unit and by whom? Does this early support consist of emotional care and confidence building, as well as attention to the physical aspects and nutritional aspects of breastfeeding?

This scenario highlights the importance of enabling mothers to recognize the cues a baby displays when ready to feed. It also emphasizes the need to provide new mothers with emotional support in addition to information about how breastfeeding works, and both are essential to provide effective breastfeeding support. Sensitive communication with a mother early after the birth of her baby can help to build her confidence and can ensure a positive start to her breastfeeding journey. Now that you are familiar with issues relating to the anatomy and physiology of breastfeeding, you should have insight into how the scenario relates to the evidence. The jigsaw model will now be used to explore the trigger scenario in more depth.

Effective communication

Effective verbal and non-verbal communication is essential when supporting women with infant feeding. Emma will have had conversations with the community midwife during pregnancy about infant feeding, and this will have prepared her for the start of her feeding journey. Questions that arise from the scenario might include: What information about recognizing feeding cues did Emma receive either before or after birth before the first breastfeed? How might this information have been provided and in what format? Might Emma have discussed infant feeding choices with her partner? What balance of information might have been most helpful for Emma and her partner; would she be more likely to want to know about the health benefits of breastfeeding or how her baby might behave in the early days after birth? Do you think it is important for the midwife to respond to Emma and her partner's questions or to provide general information about infant feeding?

Woman-centred care

Information about infant feeding should be specific to the needs of the woman and her partner. Questions that arise from the scenario might include: Had Emma and/or her partner any experience of infant feeding from friends or family members? If so, was this encouraging for her? Did

Emma receive information about infant feeding that built on her existing knowledge and understanding? Were discussions about infant feeding conducted in a way that was sensitive to Emma's emotional wellbeing? Was she given the opportunity to ask questions about issues that were important to her?

Using best evidence

High resolution ultrasound studies have led to updated knowledge of the anatomy of the breast. Understanding this and the physiology underpinning the production and ejection of breast milk, as well as the way that a baby breastfeeds has potential to improve support provided for breastfeeding mothers. Questions that arise from the scenario might include: Does Emma understand that breasts are not containers of milk but that breast milk is produced constantly in small quantities when breastfeeding? Oxytocin plays a role not only in milk ejection but also in the way mothers such as Emma interact with their baby; how might you use this focus on relationship building that is advocated within the UNICEF Baby Friendly Initiative when supporting breastfeeding mothers? Is there evidence of a link between the production of oxytocin and prevention of postnatal depression?

Professional and legal issues

Midwives should always practice within the framework of their profession and the law. In this scenario, questions that need to be addressed to ensure that the woman's care fulfils statutory obligations include: Has the midwife supporting Emma been trained at least to the minimum standards set out by the UNICEF Baby Friendly Initiative? Are there local or national guidelines that relate to early breastfeeding support that Emma might require at this time? How will the midwife ensure she makes adequate time within the context of the busy postnatal ward to provide Emma with high-quality breastfeeding support? How would the midwife document care and support she provided for Emma?

Team working

Emma will have received support for infant feeding after birth within the labour ward and on the postnatal ward; both settings may involve care from a range of health professionals.

Questions that arise from the scenario might include: Who has provided Emma with breastfeeding support? How was the care provided for Emma and her baby communicated between members of the team? How and where was this care documented?

Clinical dexterity

A midwife supporting a woman to breastfeed will need an understanding of the anatomy of the breast and the physiology of breast milk production. The crucial clinical skill will be sensitive communication to enable the midwife to build on Emma's existing knowledge to provide information about how breastfeeding works in combination with emotional support. Questions that arise from the scenario might include: What do women expect from the midwife providing breastfeeding support? Is listening as important as provision of information? Can the midwife use observation of the baby's behaviour to increase Emma's knowledge and build her confidence? If so, how can this be done effectively?

Models of care

The various models of care available for birth can affect continuity of midwifery care and support for infant feeding. For example, women receiving midwife-led care in a birth centre may be supported by fewer midwives, and this is likely to enhance their ability to build effective relationships. Questions that arise from the scenario might include: Does Emma have a named midwife who is responsible for her care? Does the documentation enable all health professionals to understand Emma's support needs? How might communication between supporters be enhanced?

Safe environment

The midwife needs to ensure that she provides a safe environment that is relaxing as possible for women in her care. When a woman feels more relaxed, this is likely to enhance production of hormones such as oxytocin providing a positive start to the journey into motherhood and infant feeding. Questions that arise from the scenario might include: Is there anything the midwife can do to the environment to make it more relaxing and feel more homely for Emma? Is there sufficient privacy and time to enable Emma to express any concerns she may have? Is it possible for the midwife to sit at the same level as Emma to facilitate good communication?

Promotes health

Supporting women with infant feeding in the early days after birth provides the midwife with a unique opportunity to enhance the emotional and physical health of both the mother and her baby. Supporting women in an empowering way using good communication skills can instill confidence in mothers and help to build a good initial relationship between mother and baby that will maximize brain development as the baby grows. Questions that arise from the scenario might include: What can the midwife say to encourage Emma to build a good relationship with her baby? Will Harry benefit from plenty of physical contact and love from Emma? If so, what will this do? Are there any ways that the midwife could enhance Emma's emotional health?

Further scenarios

The following scenarios enable you to consider how specific situations influence the care the midwife provides. Use the jigsaw model to explore the issues raised in the scenario.

SCENARIO 1

Helena gave birth to a baby girl, Jessica, 5 days ago who has been breastfeeding well and frequently since birth. Helena is concerned that her partner, David, does not feel as involved as she would like and has asked the community midwife about the possibility of replacing the evening breastfeed with a bottle of formula so that David can feed this to Jessica.

Practice point

The midwife supporting Helena will need to communicate sensitively. She should ask open questions and listen carefully to Helena's responses to find out more about Helena's feelings and understanding. The midwife will then be able to build on Helena's existing knowledge to sensitively provide further evidence-based information.

Further questions specific to Scenario 1 include:
1. What effect would missing a breastfeed have on prolactin and production of breast milk?
2. If Helena did not breastfeed for one feed and did not express breast milk, what would be the action of feedback inhibitor of lactation (FIL)?
3. Is Helena aware of the effect that reducing breastfeeds will have on her production of breast milk?
4. If Helena chose to give a formula feed, would this be absorbed as easily as breast milk?
5. Are there other ways that David could be involved in Jessica's care?
6. Consider how you would discuss these issues with Helena whilst enabling her to remain in control of her infant feeding choices.

SCENARIO 2

Holly's baby, Tom, is 7 days old and is breastfeeding well now. In the first few days, Holly's nipples felt sore and she had support from her midwife to ensure that Tom was feeding effectively. Now she is at home and her mother-in-law who is staying to help with the new baby expects Tom to settle for long periods and has been telling Holly she will 'spoil him' if she keeps cuddling him. However, Holly feels she has simply been responding to Tom's feeding cues.

Practice point

Mothers, like Holly, instinctively respond to their baby's needs and it is not possible to 'spoil' a young baby. By responding to Tom's needs and cuddling him, Holly is optimizing Tom's brain development; this responsiveness will also enable him to feed often, ensuring high levels of oxytocin and prolactin that will ultimately help Holly to establish and maintain her milk supply.

Further questions specific to Scenario 2 include:

1. How might the midwife reassure Holly about building a relationship with Tom? What online resources might you make her aware of?
2. Do you think the midwife would want to observe Holly's baby feeding? If so, what might be gained from doing this?
3. What might the midwife discuss with Holly about the relationship with her baby and brain development?
4. How could the midwife tactfully approach this situation to maintain relations between Holly and her mother-in-law?
5. How might the midwife enlist the support of Holly's mother-in-law?
6. Do you think Holly might benefit from attending a baby café or mother-to-mother support group? If so, how might the midwife discuss this with Holly?

Conclusion

Breastfeeding is the optimum nutrition for babies, but it is much more than that as it involves emotions and confidence. Mothers often feel uncertain at this time and may need information to understand what to do and confirmation that they are doing well. Midwives have an important role to play by providing women with enough evidence-based information of the anatomy and physiology of breastfeeding to enable them to understand what might work. Equally important is good communication and emotional support that takes account of their individual choices in relation to infant feeding.

Resources

Best Beginnings Baby Buddy app. Available at: http://www.bestbeginnings.org.uk/baby-buddy.

Breastfeeding and relationships in the early days video. Available at: http://www.unicef.org.uk/BabyFriendly/Resources/AudioVideo/Breastfeeding-and-relationships-in-the-early-days/.

Importance of relationship building video. Available at: http://www.unicef.org.uk/BabyFriendly/Resources/Resources-for-parents/Building-a-happy-baby/.

National Institute for Health and Care Excellence (NICE 2014). Postnatal care up to 8 weeks after birth. *Clinical Guideline 37*. London: National Collaborating Centre for Primary Care.

UNICEF Baby Friendly Initiative. Building a Happy Baby leaflet. Available at: http://www.unicef.org.uk/BabyFriendly/Resources/Resources-for-parents/Building-a-happy-baby/.

References

Geddes, D.T., 2007a. The anatomy of the lactating breast: latest research and clinical implications. Infant 3, 59–63.

Geddes, D.T., 2007b. Inside the lactating breast: the latest anatomy research. J. Midwifery Womens Health 52, 556–563.

Genna, C.W., Sandora, L., 2013. Breastfeeding: normal sucking and swallowing. In: Genna, C.W. (Ed.), Supporting Suckling Skills in Breastfeeding Infants. Jones and Bartlett, London.

Health and Social Care Information Centre, 2012. Infant Feeding Survey 2010. Health and Social Care Information Centre, London.

Pollard, M., 2012. Evidence-Based Care for Breastfeeding Mothers. Routledge, London.

Ramsey, D.T., Kent, R.A., Hartmann, R.A., Hartmann, P.E., 2005. Anatomy of the lactating human breast redefined with ultrasound imaging. J. Anat. 206, 525–534.

UNICEF Baby Friendly Initiative UK, 2014. The UNICEF UK Baby Friendly Initiative Training Pack. UNICEF Baby Friendly Initiative UK, London.

Uvnas-Moberg, K., Petersson, M., 2005. Oxytocin, a mediator of anti-stress, well-being, social interaction, growth and healing. Z. Psychosom. Med. Psychother. 51, 57–80.

Wambach, K., Riordan, J., 2015. Breastfeeding and Human Lactation. Jones and Bartlett, London.

CHAPTER 4

Skin-to-skin contact after birth

TRIGGER SCENARIO

Rosie has just given birth to her first baby 2 days after her due date. Her healthy baby boy, Tom, cried for a short while immediately after birth and is now lying prone on Rosie's chest. Tom has been relaxed and sleepy since the birth but is now, 30 minutes later, becoming more awake and is starting to look around. He looks at Rosie's right nipple and pushes his head up and moves it from side-to-side murmuring slightly as he does so. Rosie looks down at him, strokes his back and talks softly to him.

Introduction

In the UK in the 1970s and 1980s, following the move to hospital birth, it was common for mothers and babies to have limited contact in the first hours after birth. Skin-to-skin contact is beneficial for all mothers and babies as there is increasing evidence that a lack of time spent in uninterrupted skin-to-skin contact both immediately after birth and beyond can deprive mothers and babies of immediate and long-lasting physical and emotional benefits (Bergman 2013). Mothers are more likely to breastfeed in the first 1 to 4 months when they have had early skin-to-skin contact and tend to breastfeed for longer (Moore et al 2012). This chapter outlines the risks associated with not enabling women and babies to spend time in skin-to-skin contact; considers a baby's behaviour when lying skin-to-skin with his mother immediately after birth; the barriers that may occur to deny women and babies this opportunity and the ways in which skin-to-skin can enhance women's breastfeeding experience later on.

UNICEF Baby Friendly Maternity standards

The following are the maternity standards that are most relevant to this chapter:

- Support all mothers and babies to initiate a close relationship and feeding soon after birth
- Enable mothers to get breastfeeding off to a good start

The risks of not enabling women and babies time in skin-to-skin contact

In all mammals, close contact between mother and baby is the norm, so it seems relevant to discuss the risks of not making this possible for all women and babies. Babies separated from their mother show signs of stress; their heart rate and respiratory rate is higher, their blood glucose levels are lower, their blood pressure increases and they cry in short bursts, which has been interpreted as a distress cry (Bergman 2013). The touch, warmth and smell of the baby when in skin-to-skin contact causes the release of oxytocin in the mother which not only increases uterine contraction and milk ejection but also reduces stress following the birth and encourages bonding between mother and baby (Uvnas-Moberg & Petersson 2005). It therefore follows that mothers who do not experience skin-to skin contact have lower levels of oxytocin and are likely to be more stressed, experience more blood loss and reduced 'let down' of colostrum. Oxytocin also raises the skin temperature of the mother's breasts which helps to keep the baby warm as it adapts to extra-uterine life. Skin-to-skin contact has also been shown to improve immunity throughout the baby's first year of life.

Babies behaviour when lying skin-to-skin with their mother after birth

When a naked baby is placed prone on his mother's bare abdomen or chest, this is referred to as *skin-to-skin contact*. Healthy newborn babies left for a long period (at least an hour) of uninterrupted time in skin-to-skin contact with their mothers immediately after birth display an inborn

Table 4.1: **Identified behaviours whilst skin-to-skin**

Phase	Behaviour
1. Birth cry	Intense crying immediately after birth
2. Relaxation	No activity of head, arms or body
3. Awakening	Small thrusts of head, up, down, from side-to-side
4. Active	Moves head and limbs without moving body, rooting activity
5. Crawling	Pushing which moves body
6. Resting	Rests with some activity such as sucking on hands
7. Familiarization	Infants has reached areola/nipple with mouth, brushing and licking
8. Suckling	Infant starts to suckle
9. Sleeping	Infant has closed its eyes

Adapted from (Widström et al 2011).

sequential pattern of behaviour. Most babies pass through nine different phases (see Table 4.1).

This sequence of behaviour relies on a number of reflexes, such the stepping-crawling reflex and the rooting reflex, and once a baby reaches the breast and starts to feed, the sucking and swallowing reflexes are important. Babies use a range of senses to find their way to the breast, but it is thought that odour cues are the most important – particularly the smell of the mother's nipple and later on the smell of the mother's milk (Widström et al 2011).

The time that babies take to self-attach to the breast is variable. If left undisturbed after birth and if the mother has not received opiates during labour most babies will attach to the breast around 55 minutes after birth, although it can take some babies considerably longer than this. In one study, some babies took 45 minutes to attach after reaching the breast (Widström et al 2011).

Activity

What evidence might you discuss with women before birth to raise awareness of the importance of skin-to-skin contact? How might you help women to incorporate this into their birth plans?

Newborn babies are vulnerable during the period of time immediately after birth when they are making the transition to extra-uterine life. At birth, the newborn is extremely sensitive to stimuli. The nerve fibres of smell and touch are connected to the seat of emotional memory, and conditioning in the brain and stimulation from contact will 'fire and wire' the infant's brain, setting the basis for vital pathways that have life-long effects on a child's emotional wellbeing (Bergman 2013). Therefore skin-to-skin contact is important for all women and babies not only those who plan to breastfeed.

A baby should be dried and covered across their back with a warmed dry towel whilst lying on the mother skin-to-skin. Mother and baby should not be left alone at this time as the mother may be very tired following birth. The midwife should monitor the condition of the mother and baby for the first few hours after birth to ensure all is well as the baby makes the transition to extra-uterine life (Entwistle 2013). As a baby is making his way to the breast, it is important not to interrupt the sequence of events because, if this happens, the baby cannot continue where he left off but will have to start again from the beginning (UNICEF Baby Friendly Initiative UK 2014). Helping a baby to attach to the breast at this time may seem helpful, but this may be counterproductive as it can lead to the baby having problems attaching and breastfeeding effectively in the future.

Activity

Access your trust infant feeding policy. What is the guidance relating to skin-to-skin immediately after birth? Does this always happen in your unit? Search for useful video clips demonstrating the behaviour of the baby whilst in skin-to-skin contact that you might recommend to women.

Barriers to skin-to-skin contact in the hospital setting

There are many reasons why mothers who give birth in the hospital setting do not spend time in skin-to-skin contact with their baby (Entwistle 2013). These may relate to routines of care, for example, weighing, examining or bathing the baby after birth; the mother needing suturing and/or wanting a wash. Other reasons may include a busy labour ward where the room is needed for another woman or the belief that the baby will get cold.

If a woman has opiates for pain relief during labour, these cross the placenta and lodge in the lipid tissue in the fetal brain affecting the central nervous system, and this often impacts on the baby's ability to crawl to the breast and to breastfeed effectively (Smith & Kroeger 2010). The paediatric half-life of drugs is much longer than the adult half-life meaning the active components of drugs remain in the baby's system, often for many hours (Smith & Kroeger 2010).

> **Activity**
>
> Consider routines of care in the period immediately after birth in your unit. How might these be changed/improved/altered to optimize the opportunity for women and babies to have protected time together in skin-to-skin contact? Find out the length of time drugs used in your unit are likely to affect babies after birth.

Skin-to-skin contact later on

Close contact between mother and baby continues to be beneficial for both mother and baby as they develop a relationship. It may be that women find a 'laid-back' breastfeeding position is a natural extension to this, and women often find this a more comfortable feeding position or a useful alternative to more traditional ways of feeding (Colson et al 2008). Skin-to skin contact can be a useful way to solve some of the challenges breastfeeding women encounter in the early days, such as breast refusal or a sleepy baby who is reluctant to feed. Fathers too can hold their baby skin-to-skin, but this should be in addition to – not instead of – skin-to-skin contact with the mother.

REFLECTION ON THE TRIGGER SCENARIO

Look back at the trigger scenario:

> Rosie has just given birth to her first baby 2 days after her due date. Her healthy baby boy, Tom, cried for a short while immediately after birth and is now lying prone on Rosie's chest. Tom has been relaxed and sleepy since the birth but is now, 30 minutes later, becoming more awake and is starting to look around. He looks at Rosie's right nipple and pushes his head up and moves it from side-to-side murmuring slightly as he does so. Rosie looks down at him, strokes his back and talks softly to him.

Tom has reached stage 4 of the sequence of behaviours babies go through when in skin-to-skin contact with their mothers. He is responding to the stimuli of touch and smell and is starting to locate his mother's nipple. This will be stimulating a hormonal response in Rosie's body. She will experience raised levels of oxytocin that will not only have a calming effect on her but will elicit maternal feelings of love and affection towards Tom. Rosie is aware of the calming effect this contact has on him after the birth and looks in wonder as he gazes up at her. What can you do to ensure that this can happen for all mothers?

Now that you are familiar with the baby's innate behaviour when lying skin-to-skin with the mother and the importance of this for ensuring a good start to the mother-baby relationship, you should have insight into how the scenario relates to the evidence. The jigsaw model will now be used to explore the trigger scenario in more depth.

Effective communication

It is essential that midwives communicate effectively with women about infant feeding before the birth of the baby, and this should include discussions about the importance of close contact early after birth. Skin-to-skin contact between Rosie and Tom after birth will reduce stress, enhance oxytocin production and start to build a positive relationship between them. Questions that arise from the scenario might include: Did the midwife discuss skin-to-skin with Rosie during antenatal appointments? If so, when did she receive this and in what format? Did this information build on Rosie's existing knowledge and understanding? Did the midwife caring for Rosie during early labour discuss Rosie's wishes during the period of time immediately after birth? Had Rosie recorded this in her birth plan?

Woman-centred care

A sensitive, individualized approach to care is essential to enable women to make choices about the care of their baby. Rosie's and Tom's needs should be prioritized over the needs of their carers or the institution. Questions that arise from the scenario might include: What does Rosie understand about the effects of early skin-to-skin contact and ongoing physical contact between her and Tom? How might you build on this knowledge to explain the effect on Tom's brain development and future wellbeing? Are there any institutional practices that might interfere with Rosie's wish for a prolonged period of time in uninterrupted skin-to-skin contact with Tom immediately after birth?

Using best evidence

A better understanding of neuroscience in recent years has meant that practices, such as separation of mothers and babies immediately after birth for routine procedures such as weighing, are not evidence-based and are therefore not justified. It is likely that separation at this time may result in harmful effects with consequences for the baby throughout his life. Questions that arise from the scenario might include: Is there any evidence that babies need to be weighed within the first hour after birth? Does prolonged uninterrupted skin-to-skin contact between mother and baby after birth increase the likelihood that babies will breastfeed spontaneously and be breastfeeding exclusively at hospital discharge? Why do babies in skin-to-skin contact with their mothers maintain their temperature?

Professional and legal issues

Midwives must practice within a professional and legal framework to maintain high standards of care and protect women and babies from potential harm. The professional standards of practice outlined in The Code (NMC 2015) require midwives to practice in line with the best available evidence and to act in the best interests of people at all times. In this scenario, questions that need to be addressed to ensure that care fulfils statutory obligations include: Has the midwife supporting Rosie been educated at least to the minimum standards set out by the UNICEF Baby Friendly Initiative? Are there local or national guidelines that relate to care in the first hour after birth? Are these evidence-based? How would the midwife document care and support she provided for Rosie and Tom?

Team working

The midwife may be responsible for the care of the mother and baby immediately after birth, but she will be supported by other members of a multi-disciplinary team. She should aim to advocate for the mother and support her decisions for care of her baby whilst maintaining good working relationships with team members. Questions that arise from the scenario might include: How will the midwife ensure parents are not disturbed as they spend time with their baby after birth? In a busy hospital labour ward setting, what factors might arise that may threaten this special time? Is there an audit of whether mothers have received skin-to-skin care for at least an hour after birth?

Clinical dexterity

In this scenario, the skill lies in not doing anything except ensuring the mother and baby are provided with privacy and time. The baby needs to take his time to explore, to allow the innate behaviours to happen. The midwife should not to be tempted to assist the baby to breastfeed as this will ultimately be counterproductive, causing problems with breastfeeding later on. Questions that arise from the scenario might include: What reflexes will come into play as Tom crawls to Rosie's breast and breastfeeds? What effect is a laid-back position likely to have at this time? Why is it important to enable Rosie and Tom to have skin-to-skin time immediately after birth rather than a few hours later?

Models of care

Women can choose to have their baby in a range of settings, such as a hospital, a birth centre or at home, and the place of birth may affect how relaxed they feel and their ability to express their wishes. For example, a woman giving birth at home or in a homely environment is more likely to feel at ease, which can affect her mothering responses in this critical period after birth. Questions that arise from the scenario might include: Where did Rosie give birth? How might the midwife adapt the environment to ensure that Rosie is as relaxed as possible after giving birth to Tom? How might the midwife ensure Rosie is provided with adequate privacy and uninterrupted time in skin-to-skin contact with Tom?

Safe environment

It is crucial to ensure the safety of mother and baby post-birth. There are not any known harmful outcomes of skin-to-skin contact; however, there have been some incidences of neonatal death whilst a baby is in skin-to-skin contact. It is therefore important to monitor the baby's condition and position to ensure maintenance of the baby's airways. Partners may be present and may have a role to play to ensure that the baby remains safe. It is essential for the midwife to achieve a balance between the need to ensure privacy but at the same time provide care immediately after birth. Questions that arise from the scenario might include: How can the midwife ensure Rosie is positioned to maximize the safety of the baby during skin-to-skin contact? How might the midwife involve Rosie's partner in this time immediately after birth? Should Rosie and her baby be left alone at this time?

Promotes health

Facilitating women to have time in skin-to-skin contact with their baby immediately after birth provides the foundation for a positive relationship, and this will directly affect the development of the baby's brain, ultimately promoting health and wellbeing. Throughout the childbirth continuum, midwives have many opportunities to discuss the importance of encouraging ongoing close contact between mother and baby and can dispel myths such as the belief that cuddling a baby will spoil him. Questions that arise from the scenario might include: How can the midwife encourage Rosie to respond to Tom's behaviour? What messages can the midwife convey to Rosie's partner?

Further scenarios

The following scenarios enable you to consider how specific situations influence the care the midwife provides. Use the jigsaw model to explore the issues raised in each situation.

Jessica is in the first stage of labour and has been experiencing strong contractions. Sally, the midwife caring for Jessica, has involved the doctor because there have been signs of fetal distress. A decision has just been made that Jessica should have a caesarean section under epidural anaesthesia. Jessica has given her consent for this but is concerned that she will not be able to have skin-to-skin contact with her baby immediately after birth.

Practice point

The UNICEF Baby Friendly Initiative recommends that all babies should have immediate skin-to-skin contact after vaginal birth and as soon as the mother is alert and responsive after a caesarean section (UNICEF Baby Friendly Initiative UK 2014). As Jessica is having a caesarean section under epidural anaesthesia, there is no reason why she should not have immediate skin-to-skin contact with her baby in theatre. A recent review of studies investigating skin-to-skin contact after caesarean section found that benefits include: physiological stability of the newborn, improved emotional wellbeing of the mother and infant and increased communication between them, possible reduction in maternal pain and improved breastfeeding outcomes (Stevens et al 2014).

Further points specific to Scenario 1 include:

1. As women who have had a caesarean section will have less circulating oxytocin, do you think that skin-to-skin contact in theatre is more or less important for this group of women?
2. Is there any evidence that women who give birth by caesarean section are less likely to initiate breastfeeding and experience more difficulties establishing breastfeeding?
3. Is skin-to-skin contact in theatre following a caesarean section common practice in the unit where you work?
4. What might be the barriers and facilitators to achieving skin-to-skin contact between mother and baby after caesarean section in your unit?
5. Who might you liaise with to ensure that Jessica's wish to have skin-to-skin with her baby is realized?
6. Do you think that extra staff will be needed to facilitate skin-to-skin contact in theatre in your unit?
7. Are there additional risks for babies immediately after birth following a caesarean section and, if so, how would you ensure you minimize these whilst the baby was in skin-to-skin contact with his mother?

Teresa has just given birth to her baby, Annie, who is currently lying peacefully on Teresa's abdomen. Annie's father, Paul, is looking on in wonder at his perfectly formed new baby and he says, 'I wonder how much she weighs?'

Practice point

A Cochrane review of 34 studies involving 2177 mothers and babies has shown that babies receiving skin-to-skin contact interact more with their mothers and cry less and that mothers are more likely to be breastfeeding in the first 1 to 4 months and to breastfeed for longer (Moore et al 2012). When babies are separated from their mothers, they display signs of distress; their heart rate, respiratory rate and blood pressure all increase. Many routine labour ward practices can interrupt the natural responses of mothers and babies in skin-to-skin contact with long-lasting detrimental consequences.

Further points specific to Scenario 2 include:

1. Look again at the behaviours identified in Table 4.1. What phase do you think Annie is currently going through?
2. Do you think it is important for Annie to be weighed at this time?
3. How might you discuss the importance of skin-to-skin contact and the nature of the critical period after birth with Paul?
4. If you were the midwife caring for Teresa, Annie and Paul, what would you say to enable you to maximize the health and wellbeing in line with The Code (NMC 2015)?
5. What evidence might you draw upon to support your discussion?
6. Is there a protocol in your unit relating to skin-to-skin contact and, if so, is it evidence-based?
7. Can you anticipate labour ward practices that are likely to interfere with skin-to-skin contact immediately after birth, and are there actions you can take to protect women and babies?

Conclusion

There are many benefits to mothers and babies of having skin-to-skin contact after birth and no known harmful effects. Despite this, it is still not common practice in all maternity units in the UK. Midwives have an important role to play in educating women of the risks of not spending time in skin-to-skin contact with their baby, whether or not they intend to breastfeed, and acting as advocates for women within labour ward environments. It is also important that women realize the potential impact that the use of pharmacological pain relief during labour can have on their baby after birth and the effect of this on infant feeding.

Resources

Biological Nurturing. *Laid back breastfeeding website*. Available at: http://www.biologicalnurturing.com/.

Bergman N. *Skin-to-skin contact*. Available at: http://www.skintoskincontact.com/dr-bergman.aspx.

Entwistle FM (2013). *The evidence and rationale for the UNICEF UK Baby Friendly Initiative standards*. UNICEF UK. Available at: http://www.unicef.org.uk/Documents/Baby_Friendly/Research/baby_friendly_evidence_rationale.pdf.

National Institute for Health and Care Excellence (2014). Postnatal care up to 8 weeks after birth. *Clinical Guideline 37*. London: National Collaborating Centre for Primary Care.

UNICEF Baby Friendly Initiative. *The first breastfeed video clip*. Available at: http://www.unicef.org.uk/BabyFriendly/Resources/AudioVideo/First-breastfeed/.

Uvnas-Moberg K (2011). *The oxytocin factor: Tapping the hormone of calm, love and healing*. London: Pinter and Martin.

References

Bergman, N., 2013. Breastfeeding and perinatal neuroscience. In: Watson Genna, C. (Ed.), Supporting Sucking Skills in Breastfeeding Infants, second ed. Jones and Bartlett, Burlington.

Colson, S.D., Meek, J.H., Hawdon, J.M., 2008. Optimal positions for the release of primitive neonatal reflexes stimulating breastfeeding. Early Hum. Dev. 84, 441–449.

Entwistle, F.M., 2013. The Evidence and Rationale for the UNICEF UK Baby Friendly Initiative Standards. UNICEF UK.

Moore, E.R., Anderson, G.C., Bergman, N., Dowswell, T., 2012. Early skin-to-skin contact for mothers and their healthy newborn infants. Cochrane Database Syst. Rev. (5), Art. No.: CD003519, doi:10.1002/14651858.CD003519.pub3.

NMC, 2015. The Code: Professional Standards of Practice and Behaviour for Nurses and Midwives. Nursing and Midwifery Council, London. Available at: https://www.nmc.org.uk/globalassets/sitedocuments/nmc-publications/nmc-code.pdf.

Smith, L.J., Kroeger, M., 2010. Impact of Birthing Practices on Breastfeeding. Jones and Bartlett, London.

Stevens, J., Schmied, V., Burns, E., Dahlen, H., 2014. Immediate or early skin-to-skin contact after a Caesarean section: a review of the literature. Matern. Child Nutr. 10, 456–473.

UNICEF Baby Friendly Initiative UK, 2014. The UNICEF UK Baby Friendly Initiative Train the Trainer. UNICEF Baby Friendly Initiative UK, London.

Uvnas-Moberg, K., Petersson, M., 2005. Oxytocin, a mediator of anti-stress, well-being, social interaction, growth and healing. Z. Psychosom. Med. Psychother. 51, 57–80.

Widström, A.M., Lilja, G., Aaltomaa-Michalias, P., et al., 2011. Newborn behaviour to locate the breast when skin-to-skin: a possible method for enabling early self-regulation. Acta Paediatr. 100, 79–85.

CHAPTER 5

Skills to support infant feeding

TRIGGER SCENARIO

Jenny looked down at her 8-day-old baby, David, who was sleeping peacefully. 'I must be doing something wrong', she thought to herself, 'otherwise why would he be feeding for such a long time and so often?' She heard a knock at the door and went to greet Amanda, the community midwife. Jenny had called to ask if the community midwife could visit because she was worried that breastfeeding was not going so well. She was not sore, but she was now becoming concerned about how often he was feeding and she felt exhausted. As they walked back into the lounge chatting, David started to wriggle, suck on his fist and began to murmur. Jenny lifted him up and holding him close said, 'And now he is wanting another feed'.

Introduction

Most women in the UK choose to breastfeed their babies, but many do not continue for as long as they would have liked (McAndrew et al 2012). There are multiple reasons why women face challenges with breastfeeding and do not find it as easy as they anticipated. Many women have never seen a baby breastfeeding, and this lack of embodied knowledge has over the years led to a loss of practical skills. The changing role of women and working away from the home since the industrial era has led to women being separated from their babies and motherhood being hidden from the public gaze (Palmer 2009). Additionally, advances in science and technology have led to safer formula feeding to the point where it is often believed to be equivalent to breastfeeding. This is not the case as formula is not a complex living fluid containing antibodies, hormones and enzymes that enhance the health of the baby.

Whilst midwives and other health professionals must support women's choices in relation to infant feeding, they have a responsibility to ensure that women have up-to-date information in order to make these choices (NMC 2015). As breastfeeding should be considered to be the normal way to feed babies, it may be useful to think about the risks of not breastfeeding (rather than the benefits of breastfeeding) for mother and baby. In developed countries, babies who are not breastfed are at increased risk of a range of problems including: gastrointestinal infection, otitis media, high blood pressure, overweight and obesity and necrotizing enterocolitis, and mothers have an increased risk of getting breast and ovarian cancer, and type 2 diabetes (Hoddinott et al 2008; Victora et al 2016). To maximize the health of mothers and babies worldwide, the World Health Organization (WHO) has recommended exclusive breastfeeding for 6 months and continuing to give some breast milk up to 2 years of age (WHO 2003). However, few women in the UK achieve this even if this is their intention, and women have reported feeling unsupported in the postnatal period (Dykes 2005).

UNICEF Baby Friendly Maternity standards

The following are the maternity standards that are most relevant to this chapter:
- Enable mothers to get breastfeeding off to a good start
- Support parents to have a close and loving relationship with their baby

UNICEF Baby Friendly UK University learning outcomes

The following are the learning outcomes that are achieved within this chapter. By the end of their midwifery education programme, students will:
- Be able to apply their knowledge and understanding of the physiology of lactation to support women to get breastfeeding off to a good start
- Be able to apply their knowledge of physiology and the principle of reciprocity to support mothers to keep their babies close and respond to their cues for feeding and comfort
- Have the knowledge and skills to support mothers and babies to continue to breastfeed as long as they want to
- Have the knowledge and skills to access the evidence that underpins infant feeding practice
- Be able to apply their knowledge of effective communication to initiate sensitive, mother-centred conversations with pregnant women and new mothers

Teaching women how to breastfeed

Learning to breastfeed is a practical skill that has been likened to learning to dance with a partner because it depends not just on one person learning it but two people getting it right at the same time (Renfrew et al 2004). As many mothers are aware, it is also a skill that must be learned quickly because it is life-giving for the baby. However, women sometimes describe feeling pressure to breastfeed and guilty if they choose not to do so (Hoddinott et al 2012). It is therefore important that midwives have the skills to enable them to teach mothers how to breastfeed and to assess whether or not a baby is breastfeeding effectively in a way that is sensitive to women's feelings.

If a baby is not attached and positioned so that he can breastfeed well, this can lead to range of problems for both mother and baby, such as sore and damaged nipples, milk stasis that can lead to engorgement, blocked ducts and mastitis. Any stasis of milk will result in a build-up of feedback inhibitor of lactation (FIL), and this will reduce the production of milk. Coupled with this, a baby who is not attached well and feeding effectively is likely to feed often and for long periods of time because he will not obtain the more fatty milk that he would normally get later in the feed. This can lead to a mother losing confidence in her ability to breastfeed and/or to provide sufficient milk for her baby (UNICEF Baby Friendly Initiative UK 2014).

Attachment

Attachment is the process of the baby taking the breast into the mouth to enable breastfeeding. Babies are born with three reflexes that enable them to attach to the breast and feed. These are: the rooting reflex – where a baby turns the head and opens the mouth when something touches the cheek; the sucking reflex – when something touches the roof of the mouth, the baby sucks and draws it into the mouth and the swallowing reflex – when the mouth fills with milk, the baby swallows. Therefore healthy term babies will attach to the breast and feed using these innate behaviours.

It is important that anyone supporting breastfeeding mothers can recognize when a baby is well-attached to the breast. The main signs that a baby is attached well are listed in Table 5.1.

Although these technical aspects of recognizing good attachment and efficient milk transfer are important and can reduce the problems and challenges women encounter, it is equally important to consider a woman's concerns and emotional wellbeing. A crucial part of this is to listen to each woman and respond in a way that builds her confidence in her ability to breastfeed so that she learns how to do it herself and feels good about it.

Table 5.1: **Signs of good attachment**

Signs of good attachment at the breast
The baby's mouth is open wide with tongue beneath the breast
The baby has a large amount of breast tissue in his mouth
The baby's chin is against and indents the breast
The baby's lower lip is curled outwards and the top lip neutral
The baby's cheeks are rounded and appear full (not sucked in)
More of the mother's areola is visible above the baby's top lip than the bottom

Adapted from (UNICEF Baby Friendly Initiative UK 2014)

Activity

Watch the short video clip of a graphic of a baby attaching well at the breast at https://www.bestbeginnings.org.uk/graphic-of-a-baby-attaching-on-the-breast/067348cf-7dd7-46cb-8f8b-9ae5ddaad028.

Compare this to the graphic of how poor attachment happens and can cause nipple trauma: https://www.unicef.org.uk/babyfriendly/baby-friendly-resources/video/ineffective-attachment/.

Consider whether these clips would be useful for you to show women in your area of work. Think about the language you use when you support a woman to breastfeed; do you use non-technical language that is easy to follow and sensitive to a woman's feelings and emotional wellbeing? Search the Internet using a phrase like 'pressure to breastfeed' and read what women are saying about the support they have or have not received to help them to breastfeed.

Positioning

Positioning is how the mother holds her baby for breastfeeding. There is no right or wrong way to hold a baby for breastfeeding, and women find a range of positions that are comfortable for them. However, whatever position is adopted, there are some principles that are helpful to enable a baby to feed easily and efficiently and to ensure the mother is comfortable. These are listed in Table 5.2.

In the UK, a bottle-feeding culture exists, and women sometimes try to breastfeed holding their baby as they would if the baby was feeding from a bottle, but this does not work for breastfeeding. Using these principles can help midwives to teach women how to position their baby optimally, but this should be carried out in a way that is sensitive to a woman's

Table 5.2: **Principles of positioning**

Principles of positioning that will make breastfeeding easier
Baby's head and body in line (i.e. head not twisted to the side whilst lying on his back)
Head free so that the baby can tilt the head back to feed
Baby's body held close to mother
Before attaching to the breast, the baby's nose is level with mother's nipple
Once the baby is feeding, the position should be sustainable

Adapted from (UNICEF Baby Friendly Initiative UK 2014).

learning needs and emotional wellbeing. The position of the baby in relation to the mother will depend on the size and shape of the breast (see Fig. 5.1). Often using a doll (with a flexible neck) or a soft toy is helpful to demonstrate various positions without the need to touch the mother or baby. This can enable the mother to learn more easily. Illustrations of range of different positions can be found in several resources (e.g. Pollard 2012). It may be useful to encourage mothers to adopt a laid-back position and to have the baby skin-to-skin if the baby is reluctant to feed or is refusing the breast as this will bring all the baby's innate reflexes into play (Colson et al 2008).

> **Activity**
>
> Do you have access to a doll/soft toy to demonstrate to mothers the various ways they might hold and position their baby? You may wish to use the DVD clip at https://www.unicef.org.uk/babyfriendly/baby -friendly-resources/video/positioning-and-attachment/.

Responsive feeding

It is important to encourage women to respond to their baby to develop a sensitive and nurturing relationship (as discussed in Chapter 2), and responding to their baby's feeding cues is a key part of this. Separation and strict feeding regimes were common in the 1960s and 70s, and books are still available advocating routine and control of babies, meaning that women often receive mixed messages that can leave them uncertain of what to do and can impact on their views of themselves as 'good mothers' (Marshall et al 2007). If this results in constraints on women's instinctive nurturing behaviour, it has potential to have long-ranging negative effects on babies' emotional adaptation and ability to form relationships throughout their life course (Newman et al 2015). Therefore women may need

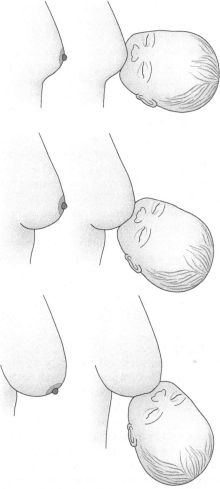

Fig. 5.1 Baby's body in relation to mother's body depending on the angle of the breast. *(From an original drawing by Hilary English.)*

information and support from the midwife to help them to recognize when their baby is ready to feed and encourage them to follow their instincts by responding to these cues.

Breastfeeding mothers should be encouraged to keep their baby close to them so that they notice the baby's feeding cues early because once the baby becomes distressed and agitated, breastfeeding becomes more difficult. Early feeding cues include the baby displaying eye movement under closed lids and becoming restless, rooting and opening the mouth. This progresses gradually, and the baby will start to move more, may stretch and wave their hands or put their fingers in their mouth. The baby may also start to make murmuring noises. Mothers should be encouraged to start to breastfeed during this time. If the baby is very agitated and crying, he may be too distressed to start feeding and will need to be calmed first. Crying is usually the last sign of a baby's hunger.

It is important to encourage the mother to develop a sensitive reciprocal relationship with her baby that includes responding to her baby's hunger cues; however, breastfeeding fulfils much more than the baby's nutritional needs. For example, it can also provide comfort and calm a distressed baby (UNICEF Baby Friendly Initiative UK 2014). The mother may also want to breastfeed if she has full breasts or wants to sit down and cuddle her baby (Entwistle 2013). Focusing on the length of time a baby breastfeeds is not usually helpful as the length of the feed may vary from baby to baby and will depend on the baby's needs at that particular time. It is important that mothers realize that breastfed babies cannot be overfed and that following their instincts to respond to their baby will not only help to ensure a plentiful milk supply but will also have long-ranging benefits to their baby's health and wellbeing.

Activity

Mothers produce colostrum in small quantities for their baby in the first few days after birth, but the small amount produced is calorie rich and contains many protective factors. Read about colostrum and note the many different protective factors and how they work.

Women are often concerned about the small quantity of colostrum. Babies are born with an excess of interstitial fluid that their body and immature kidneys must process so the concentrated nature of colostrum is helpful. Belly balls that visually display the size of a newborn's stomach can help mothers to understand the small quantities the baby needs during the first few days (Day 1: 5–7 ml, marble size; Day 3: 22–27 ml, ping pong ball size; Day 5: 57 ml, large egg size). Can you make a set of belly balls you can use in practice?

Teaching hand expression

Learning to hand express breast milk is useful for mothers because it can enable them to work out ways to solve some common breastfeeding challenges, such as blocked milk ducts or difficulties breastfeeding due to engorgement and can be empowering for mothers (UNICEF Baby Friendly Initiative UK 2014). One study concluded that women who expressed breast milk were more likely to breastfeed to 6 months (Win et al 2006). It is easy to teach and does not take long.

First, the mother should be encouraged to wash her hands with soap and water and massage the breast, either by gently rolling her fist over it or by massaging towards the nipple without dragging or pulling the breast tissue. This tactile stimulation will encourage the release of oxytocin and prolactin that will help the mother's milk to flow and increase milk production (Marshall 2012). She should be shown using a model or knitted breast how to hold the breast with her hand in a 'C' shape, to gently feel approximately 2.5 cms behind the nipple and squeeze rhythmically holding a clean container beneath the breast to catch the expressed milk. If the mother is expressing in the early days after birth, it is important to explain that colostrum will be present in small quantities and will not squirt from the breast. It may be helpful to play some relaxing music and, if separated from her baby, the mother may find that an item of clothing or a photograph of the baby helps the release of oxytocin and therefore the flow of milk or colostrum. Many mothers find hand expressing more effective than electric pumps, but this tends to depend on how they feel about it. If using an electric pump, starting with hand expression can be helpful. A recently updated Cochrane review suggests that hand expression or low-cost pumps may be as effective as large electric pumps and that an audio relaxation tape, warming the breast and massage can increase the volume of milk expressed (Becker et al 2015).

Activity

Watch the DVD clip at https://www.unicef.org.uk/babyfriendly/baby-friendly-resources/video/hand-expression/.

You may like to either knit or ask someone to knit you a breast to use as a teaching aid. A pattern can be found at http://www.lcgb.org/lcgb-knitted-breast-the-pattern/.

REFLECTION ON THE TRIGGER SCENARIO

Jenny looked down at her 8-day-old baby, David, who was sleeping peacefully. 'I must be doing something wrong', she thought to herself, 'otherwise why would he be feeding for such a long time and so often?' She heard a knock at the door and went to greet Amanda, the community midwife. Jenny had called to ask if the community midwife could visit because she was worried that breastfeeding was not going so well. She was not sore, but she was now becoming concerned about how often he was feeding and she felt exhausted. As they walked back into the lounge chatting, David started to wriggle, suck on his fist and began to murmur. Jenny lifted him up and holding him close said, 'And now he is wanting another feed'.

This scenario is based on a situation encountered in practice as part of a research study (with all names changed). Amanda listened to Jenny; she watched her baby feed and recognized that he was not properly attached and was therefore not feeding effectively. Amanda explained to Jenny that he was almost there but just needed to be a little further on and discussed the signs she should look for to know that he was attached well at the breast. Jenny later described how this had helped her: '...before she came, I was thinking, you know "I'll have to see what she says, but if, you know, if nothing comes of it then perhaps I'll have to start, I'll think about giving up"... and then once she'd been and sort of explained to me, I felt a lot more positive... and able to continue really.'

Now that you are familiar with some of the skills needed to support women who have chosen to breastfeed, you should have insight into how the scenario relates to the evidence. The jigsaw model will now be used to explore the trigger scenario in more depth.

Effective communication

Communication is a crucial element of support for breastfeeding women. It is important that the practitioner is aware of their body language, for example, sitting down to speak to Jenny rather than standing over her will help to minimize the power differential and convey the message that there is sufficient time to provide support. Women learn in different ways and many will gain more from visual as well as verbal information. Efforts should be made to ensure that Jenny understands the information being conveyed to her, and this may be achieved by encouraging her to reflect back on what she has gleaned. Questions that arise from the scenario might include: Why is it helpful for Amanda to watch David feed before offering information to Jenny? How might Amanda use what she sees as David is feeding to convey further information to Jenny? Jenny considered this episode of communication positively and felt able to continue breastfeeding; what aspects of the interaction do you think might have achieved this?

Woman-centred care

Women want support for breastfeeding that is detailed and specific to their needs at any particular point in time (Marshall et al 2007). Generalized abstract information is not considered to be as helpful. Practical help with breastfeeding is essential but so too is attention to each woman's emotional wellbeing, which often involves reassurance that they are doing it right. Questions that arise from the scenario might include: What visible signs of effective feeding might Amanda discuss with Jenny? How might Amanda involve Jenny's partner? How do you think Jenny would have felt if Amanda had said 'that's not right' rather than conveying the message that David just needed to be a little further on her breast?

Using best evidence

Midwives must ensure they are aware of the most recent good quality evidence. Cochrane reviews can provide a summary of good quality information about the effectiveness of particular interventions. For example, a Cochrane review has shown that extra support for breastfeeding women from both health professionals and peer supporters encourages them to breastfeed more exclusively and for longer (McFadden et al 2017). This support is most effective when offered proactively and delivered face-to-face rather than by telephone. Questions that arise from the scenario might include: Jenny felt able to ask the community midwife to call when she thought breastfeeding was not going so well, but do you think all women would do this? Why do you think that regular, structured support for breastfeeding women has been shown to be most effective? Might Jenny benefit from meeting other breastfeeding mothers? Do you know what support groups and breastfeeding cafes exist in your area?

Professional and legal issues

Midwives must ensure they have the relevant skills to support women with all aspects of care including infant feeding. They must also listen to mothers' preferences and concerns to enable them to respond appropriately (NMC 2015). Questions that arise from the scenario might include: How do midwives develop and maintain their skills to support women with infant feeding? Are there regular updates on infant feeding where you work? Do you reflect on support you have provided for a woman you have cared for in an effort to improve your care? What might have happened if Amanda had failed to recognize that David poorly attached and was not feeding effectively? If you had provided the support to Jenny, how would you have documented this?

Team working

The midwife works as part of a team in all aspects of maternity care including infant feeding. Many women receive support for infant feeding from peer supporters, and this can be on the postnatal ward and in the community setting. Midwives must ensure they work in partnership to help women harness help and support from a range of sources. Peer support is discussed in detail in Chapter 12. The midwife also needs to involve other family members wherever possible as some women gain much support from their family, for example, if their own mother has previously breastfed. However, family members, although they usually mean well, can make comments that cause breastfeeding mothers worry and anxiety. The midwife may have opportunities to involve and educate family particularly in the community setting. Questions that arise from the scenario might include: What might you do to ensure you build a good working relationship with peer supporters in the area where you work? How might you involve other family members when visiting a woman in the community setting? Do you think it might be useful to discuss with Jenny ways she might manage negative comments about breastfeeding from family?

Clinical dexterity

Women in Jenny's situation receiving help to breastfeed do not usually appreciate the baby being attached to the breast for them as this does not enable them to learn how to breastfeed their baby. It also tends to undermine their self-confidence, which can extend to mothering generally, as well as breastfeeding. The clinical skills Amanda needs in this case encompass both recognition of good or poor attachment and skilful effective communication. Done well, this will enable Jenny to not only learn what to do herself to breastfeed her baby effectively but also to feel good about this. Questions that arise from the scenario might include: How might Amanda explain to Jenny how a baby attaches to the breast? What visual aids might she use? Do you regularly use a knitted breast or doll to show women how a baby latches onto the breast? Do you think suggesting a laid-back position for breastfeeding might help Jenny and, if so, why?

Models of care

The model of care that a breastfeeding woman is receiving has potential to affect her perception of support and/or her ability to ask for help. For example, she may feel more comfortable to receive breastfeeding support from a known midwife. However, Jenny had not met Amanda before and yet she found the care Amanda provided to be very helpful and encouraging. This suggests that the model of care is not as important as the actual care women receive as long as the care provided is effective and sensitive. Questions that arise from the scenario might include: How would Amanda document the care she provided to ensure that Jenny's named community midwife is able to continue to offer support during subsequent visits? Are there processes in place to ensure that women in the area where you work are easily able to ask for extra support? Is there anything that might make this easier for women?

Safe environment

The midwife needs to ensure that women and babies in her care remain safe. If Amanda had failed to recognize that David was not feeding effectively, this could have resulted initially in David continuing to display unsettled behaviour and lack of weight gain and, in more extreme cases, dehydration. Routine weighing can provide a safety net to ensure that babies who are not feeding well are not overlooked, but weighing does not replace the need for the midwife to adequately assess the effectiveness of breastfeeding. A breastfeeding assessment tool that can be used by mothers and midwives is available at https://www.unicef.org.uk/babyfriendly/baby-friendly-resources/guidance-for-health-professionals/tools-and-forms-for-health-professionals/breastfeeding-assessment-tools/. Questions that arise from the scenario might include: What visual signs that David is receiving a good amount of breast milk might be assessed? How could Amanda discuss these visual signs with Jenny? Why do you think that observable and measurable signs that a baby is getting enough milk are helpful to women?

Promotes health

Most women know that breastfeeding is the method of infant feeding that will ensure optimal health for their baby, and the majority choose this (McAndrew et al 2012). However, many women stop breastfeeding before they wanted to. This is at least partially because we live in a society that does not support women to breastfeed but also because women do not always receive the practical help and emotional support they need to help them to continue. It is essential that breastfeeding support is part of holistic care for women and babies. The midwife should ensure that care and support is provided in a way that not only provides high quality physical care but also pays attention to the woman's emotional and psychological wellbeing as this can impact on her ability to develop a nurturing relationship with her baby. Questions that arise from the scenario might include: Do you think Jenny was instinctively responding to David's feeding cues? How might Amanda build on this to encourage further development of the relationship between Jenny and David? How might Amanda find out about the way comments from family members are affecting Jenny?

Further scenarios

The following scenarios enable you to consider how specific situations influence the care the midwife provides. Use the jigsaw model to explore the issues raised in each situation.

SCENARIO 1

Janette has had midwife-led care at a birth centre. Her baby Miles has been held skin-to-skin after birth, has had a breastfeed and has slept since. Janette has just woken up and noticed that Miles is wriggling, mouthing and starting to murmur. She thinks to herself 'it looks like he might need another feed'.

Practice point

Although Janette has breastfed Miles already and appears to recognize his feeding cues, it would be helpful for the midwife to reinforce this by pointing these out and to encourage Janette to feed Miles before he starts to cry. This is likely to lead to effective breastfeeding and will help to develop a positive mother/baby relationship.

Further points specific to Scenario 1 include:
1. How might the midwife caring for Janette use this opportunity to support the development of the mother/baby relationship?
2. How might the midwife explain how a baby feeds to Janette in a way that leaves her feeling able to do it herself when she goes home?
3. Once Miles is breastfeeding, what should the midwife see if he is well-attached to the breast and feeding effectively?
4. How might the midwife explain the principles of positioning to Janette?
5. What communication skills might the midwife use whilst she is helping Janette?

SCENARIO 2

Alia's baby has been breastfeeding enthusiastically. He self-attached and fed after birth, had a long sleep and then has been feeding often since. They are now preparing to go home from the postnatal ward. The midwife caring for Alia is about to explain how to hand express breast milk.

Practice Point

Ensuring women know how to hand express breast milk can empower them. This skill can be used by women to work out a solution to a range of minor breastfeeding challenges, such as a blocked milk duct. It can also be helpful for women to be able to express once breastfeeding is established to leave some breast milk for others to feed.

Further points specific to Scenario 2 include:

1. What visual aids might the midwife use to enhance her explanation of hand expression?
2. What would Alia collect her breast milk in and would it need to be sterile?
3. How long can breast milk be stored in the fridge?
4. For what length of time can breast milk be frozen?
5. How should breast milk be defrosted?
6. Can you find a leaflet from a reliable source that you could give to women?

Conclusion

Midwives have a responsibility to ensure they have the basic skills to enable them to support breastfeeding women. However, it is essential to listen to women's concerns and convey these skills to women in such a way that they gain confidence in their ability to breastfeed; that they feel supported in their efforts rather than pressurized. Effective support from midwives and other members of the maternity care team can make a real difference to women.

Resources

Breastfeeding Network. *Expressing and storing breast milk leaflet.* Available at: https://www.breastfeedingnetwork.org.uk/wp-content/pdfs/ BFNExpressing_and_Storing.pdf.

National Institute for Health and Care Excellence (2014). Postnatal care up to 8 weeks after birth. *Clinical Guideline 37.* London: National Collaborating Centre for Primary Care.

NCT. *What's in a nappy?* Available at: http://www.ouh.nhs.uk/women/maternity/ postnatal/infant-feeding/documents/nappy.pdf .

UNICEF. *Breastfeeding and relationships in the early days video.* Available at: http:// www.unicef.org.uk/BabyFriendly/Resources/AudioVideo/Breastfeeding -and-relationships-in-the-early-days/.

UNICEF. *Importance of relationship building video.* Available at: http:// www.unicef.org.uk/BabyFriendly/Resources/Resources-for-parents/ Building-a-happy-baby/.

References

Becker, G.E., Smith, H.A., Cooney, F., 2015. Methods of milk expression for lactating women. Cochrane Database Syst. Rev. (2), CD006170.

Colson, S.D., Meek, J.H., Hawdon, J.M., 2008. Optimal positions for the release of primitive neonatal reflexes stimulating breastfeeding. Early Hum. Dev. 84, 441–449.

Dykes, F., 2005. A critical ethnographic study of encounters between midwives and breastfeeding women in postnatal wards in England. Midwifery 21, 241–252.

Entwistle, F.M., 2013. The Evidence and Rationale for the UNICEF UK Baby Friendly Initiative Standards. UNICEF UK, London.

Hoddinott, P., Craig, L.C.A., Britten, J., McInnes, R.M., 2012. A serial qualitative interview study of infant feeding experiences: idealism meets realism. BMJ Open 2 (2), e000504. doi:10.1136/bmjopen-2011-000504.

Hoddinott, P., Tappin, D., Wright, C., 2008. Breast feeding. BMJ 336, 881–887.

Marshall, J., 2012. Infant feeding: Anatomy and physiology. Pract. Midwife 15, 38–41.

Marshall, J.L., Godfrey, M., Renfrew, M.J., 2007. Being a 'good mother': Managing breastfeeding and merging identities. Soc. Sci. Med. 65, 2147–2159.

McAndrew, F., Thompson, J., Fellows, L., et al., 2012. Infant Feeding Survey 2010. Health and Social Care Information Centre, London.

McFadden, A., Gavine, A., Renfrew, M.J., et al., 2017. Support for healthy breastfeeding mothers with healthy term babies. Cochrane Database Syst. Rev. (2), Art. No.: CD001141, doi:10.1002/14651858.CD001141.pub5.

Newman, L., Sivaratnam, C., Komiti, A., 2015. Attachment and early brain development - neuroprotective interventions in infant-caregiver therapy. Transl. Dev. Psychiatry 3, 28647. Available at: http://dx.doi.org/10.3402/tdp.v3.28647.

NMC, 2015. The Code: Professional Standards of Practice and Behaviour for Nurses and Midwives. Nursing and Midwifery Council, London. Available at: https://www.nmc.org.uk/globalassets/sitedocuments/nmc-publications/nmc-code.pdf.

Palmer, G., 2009. The Politics of Breastfeeding: When Breasts are Bad for Business. Pinter and Martin, London.

Pollard, M., 2012. Evidence-Based Care for Breastfeeding Mothers. Routledge, London.

Renfrew, M.J., Fisher, C., Arms, S., 2004. Bestfeeding: How to Breastfeed Your Baby, third ed. Celestial Arts, New York.

UNICEF Baby Friendly Initiative UK, 2014. The UNICEF UK Baby Friendly Initiative Train the Trainer. UNICEF Baby Friendly Initiative UK, London.

Victora, C.G., Bahl, R., Barros, A.J.D., et al., 2016. Breastfeeding in the 21st century: epidemiology, mechanisms, and lifelong effect. Lancet 387, 475–490.

Win, N., Binns, C., Zhao, Y., et al., 2006. Breastfeeding duration in mothers who express breast milk: a cohort study. Int. Breastfeed. J. 1, 28.

World Health Organisation, 2003. Global Strategy for Infant and Young Child Feeding. World Health Organisation, Geneva.

CHAPTER 6

The social context of infant feeding

TRIGGER SCENARIO

Sally has just arrived 'home' to her mother's house from the hospital with her partner Joe. They are staying with Sally's mother for a few weeks before moving into their own house. Sally had wanted to have her baby at home as she hated hospitals but had to be transferred to hospital during labour. After baby Eva was born, Sally was distraught because she did not have the opportunity to breastfeed within the first hour (she had read that this was important), but she enjoyed the 'special moment' when she finally breastfed. Sally breastfed Eva a couple of times but was then struggling and asked for help from the midwives. A range of different suggestions were offered by midwives who were very willing to help but seemed very busy. None of the suggestions seemed to help, and Sally had been left feeling confused and upset. Sally is now feeling much more relaxed at home with her mother as she is confident her mother can help if needed as she has breastfed all of her children. Sally's partner, Joe, is supportive emotionally but has already suggested Sally should give Eva a bottle of formula.

Introduction

Infant feeding is much more than simply nutrition for a baby as it has cultural and social meaning as part of motherhood (Marshall et al 2007). The choices women make in relation to infant feeding can be reinforced or constrained by social norms and expectations. Information and reactions from significant people within women's social networks (including health professionals) can affect the way they feel – their emotions, attitudes and consequently their behaviour. The huge variation in breastfeeding initiation and continuation rates across different countries provides evidence for the effect of the social and cultural context within which infant feeding takes place. For example, the infant feeding survey published in 2010 in the UK showed that, although 81% of women started to breastfeed, only 40% of those who started were still breastfeeding at all when the baby is 6 months old (McAndrew et al 2012). Whereas in Norway, although a similar percentage of women start to breastfeed (81.7%), 80% of them are still breastfeeding at 6 months (Häggkvist et al 2010).

The social environment in which people live shapes knowledge and the meaning given to infant feeding practices and other aspects of motherhood. This happens at a range of different levels – societal, immediate social networks and individual or family influences. A better understanding of the family situation and social network within which a mother is feeding her baby can help midwives and other health professionals to support her more appropriately. Rather than simply conveying 'breast is best' style messages that can be perceived as 'pressure' to breastfeed, women may want help to find strategies to manage negative comments from family and friends or ways to find supportive breastfeeding allies.

UNICEF Baby Friendly Maternity standards

The following are the maternity standards that are most relevant to this chapter:
- Support pregnant women to recognize the importance of breastfeeding and early relationships for the health and well-being of their baby.

UNICEF Baby Friendly UK University learning outcomes

The following are the learning outcomes that are achieved within this chapter. By the end of their midwifery education programme, students will:
- Have an understanding of infant feeding culture within the UK and the various influences and constraints of women's infant feeding decisions
- Have the knowledge and skills to support mothers and babies to continue to breastfeed for as long as they want to
- Be able to apply their knowledge of effective communication to initiate sensitive, mother-centred conversations with pregnant women and new mothers
- Have the knowledge and skills to access the evidence that underpins infant feeding practice

---

Support for breastfeeding mothers

Mothers can receive support from a range of different sources, such as health professionals or lay/peer supporters and from their family and informal social networks. A Cochrane review drawing on data involving more than 74,000 women from 29 countries found that extra support provided by either lay supporters or professionals or both helped women to continue to breastfeed for longer and helped them to exclusively breastfeed for longer (McFadden et al 2017). Face-to-face support had more effect than telephone support (McFadden et al 2017). Schmied et al (2011) carried out a metasynthesis of qualitative research papers to examine the components of support that women felt were important. They found that building rapport and a trusting relationship and 'being there' for each woman were key components, making them feel relaxed and comfortable rather than pressurized by feeling rushed by busy supporters. Within a trusting relationship and given time, women felt much more able to ask questions. The same review also suggested that many women lack confidence and appreciate supporters who acknowledge how they are feeling and tell them when they are doing okay – that is, they offer timely support appropriate to the woman's needs (Schmied et al 2011).

A style of support that is facilitative and provides women with realistic information is appreciated, including practical and personal aspects of breastfeeding – accurate information with sufficient detail (Schmied et al 2011). Rather than oversimplified advice given in a didactic style, women often want a discursive two-way exchange with practical help where they are shown rather than told and often they want to know why a suggestion might work to make sense of the situation.

Activity

Active listening is an important skill to use when supporting women to breastfeed. Using an Internet search engine, enter the words 'active listening quiz', choose one and use it to assess your active listening skills. How might this help you to support breastfeeding women? Do you always use open questions to encourage dialogue with women?

Infant feeding is a key part of the transition to motherhood, and the support women need changes over time as they make this transition. It is therefore useful to consider this chronologically to explore that different factors have impact at different times in the infant feeding journey and the role of the midwife within this.

Pregnancy and decisions about infant feeding

During pregnancy, women generally receive the message 'breast is best' whether this is from attending antenatal education sessions or from reading books or magazines. Midwives can play a significant role in the promotion of breastfeeding either when seeing women in antenatal clinics or when delivering antenatal education sessions. As discussed in Chapter 2, antenatal education should include preparation for the transition to parenthood rather than simply promotion of the health benefits of breastfeeding (Barlow et al 2009). Whilst women usually expect health professionals to promote breastfeeding, this can sometimes be perceived as 'pressure' to breastfeed particularly if significant people in the mother's life are either ambivalent or unsupportive of the mother's decision to breastfeed (Marshall & Godfrey 2012). Research carried out in Scotland has suggested that women do not feel the antenatal information they receive prepares them well – that the reality is very different (Hoddinott et al 2012). Murphy (1999) discusses the strong moral nature of infant feeding decisions and suggests that the statements women make during pregnancy are predictive of whether or not they will initiate breastfeeding. However, such decisions are complex and are influenced by partners or the way the mother's own mother breastfed, and can be affected positively or negatively by seeing others breastfeed or hearing stories about their experiences (Hoddinott & Pill 1999).

Activity

Consider how women in your area of work are introduced to breastfeeding. Is there opportunity for women to discuss their experiences and beliefs? Are visual experiences of a baby breastfeeding or discussions with a breastfeeding woman part of this?

Breastfeeding in the early days

Many women feel vulnerable and uncertain in the early days after birth, and breastfeeding is often a major factor within this. Women often want to know they are 'doing it right' or to have ways of knowing that things are going well such as the baby feeding well and being content (Marshall & Godfrey 2012). In the hospital setting, there is potential for midwives to support women with both the emotional and practical aspects of breastfeeding. However, time and structural constraints in the medicalized postnatal ward setting can mean that midwives are unable to build relationships with women and care can become routine, meaning that contact with breastfeeding women becomes disjointed (Dykes 2006).

Women can have mixed feelings about going home from the hospital, especially if they have encountered challenges breastfeeding. They are often excited to be going home but at the same time can be concerned because they recognize that professional help will not be so easily available. Building confidence at this time is crucial, particularly with the practical and technical skills of breastfeeding, but the emotional aspects are equally important (Marshall et al 2007).

Activity

Consider your last interaction with a breastfeeding woman. Did you use open questions to encourage the woman to talk about how she was feeling? Consider the way you offer help to breastfeeding women. Do you always explain why you are offering a particular suggestion so that she can work it out herself next time? Do you involve partners in these interactions? Read or listen to the mixed feelings women have about going home at http://www.healthtalkonline.org/Pregnancy_children/ Breastfeeding.

Continuing to breastfeed

Later in their breastfeeding experience, women often become concerned about whether or not the baby is getting enough milk. Ways that women can 'know' that their baby is getting enough milk include the following: the baby appearing healthy and having wet and dirty nappies, the way their breasts feel before and after a feed, their ability to express milk and the baby gaining weight. These can be considered to be ways of making the invisible visible and can increase women's confidence, but a range of factors can undermine this confidence (Marshall et al 2007). People in women's social networks often make comments about babies' behaviour that cause women to question their ability to provide sufficient milk for their baby. Group-based peer support for breastfeeding mothers as provided at many Children's Centres or Baby Bistros can help and is popular with mothers because this normalizes breastfeeding in a relaxed social environment that helps improve wellbeing (Hoddinott et al 2006).

Activity

Where can breastfeeding women find mother-to-mother support in a group setting in your area? If you were to facilitate such a group, how might you consider alleviating anxieties a mother might have when attending for the first time?

Providing culturally sensitive infant feeding support

Culture can be considered to be the beliefs, norms, values and rules of behaviour of a particular group that are shared and that guide thinking and decisions (Wambach 2016). Culture is rather like the unwritten rules that we all follow and often unconsciously constrains behaviour and actions. To take account of the cultural situation within which women live, it is important that midwives and others who provide support to mothers are sensitive to their individual situation and needs. These may or may not vary across women's individual characteristics such as age, social, cultural or ethnic background. As discussed earlier, asking open questions and listening carefully to women will lead to the provision of culturally sensitive care through exploration of women's expectations of support.

Women from minority ethnic groups are more likely to start breastfeeding and to continue for longer but they are less likely to breastfeed exclusively than the majority population (McAndrew et al 2012). However, sometimes women from minority ethnic groups receive poor quality support, and there can be a range of reasons for this, such as poor communication and stereotyping. A qualitative study within which 23 women of Bangladeshi origin were interviewed and focus groups were conducted with 28 health practitioners found that many of the breastfeeding support needs of Bangladeshi women were similar to the needs of the majority population and some were different. This study showed that, for example, the need for proactive, practical support for positioning and attachment and reassurance that they will produce enough milk for their baby is common for all women regardless of ethnicity (McFadden et al 2012a). Cultural factors did make a difference to breastfeeding women in some ways, for example, women having household responsibilities, having to breastfeed in private within their home and the influence of grandmothers. However, women's household circumstances varied considerably, and this was not recognized by practitioners who tended to stereotype women as passive (McFadden et al 2012a). When midwives and other health practitioners make such assumptions, the support provided is unlikely to meet women's needs.

A key point is that midwives should provide holistic care to women and their families and within this to ensure they respond to cultural differences sensitively. One important misconception is that women of Asian descent do not feed their babies colostrum and will therefore feed their babies formula during the first few days of life. McFadden et al (2012b) explored this issue from the perspectives of Bangladeshi mothers, grandmothers and health practitioners and found that Bangledeshi mothers and grandmothers may doubt the adequacy of colostrum especially when difficulties were experienced with starting to breastfeed in the early feeds after birth. However, these concerns were reinforced by routine use of formula that led to the expectation that formula would be given. Interestingly, the women in this study who were cared for in hospitals with BFI accreditation did not feed their babies formula (McFadden et al 2012b).

Similar misconceptions can also occur in relation to young mothers and mothers from disadvantaged groups. Successive surveys in the UK and other developed countries demonstrate that younger women are least likely to choose to breastfeed and, if they do, are likely to stop sooner. Young mothers often encounter dilemmas about infant feeding. They tend to know that 'breast is best', and internalize the moral idea that 'good mothers' will breastfeed, but for many breastfeeding is not their social norm. They may not have seen mothers breastfeeding, and it may not be their culturally expected behaviour (Poole & Gephart 2014). Young mothers whose own mothers breastfed are more likely to choose to breastfeed and to continue for longer. Other challenges for young mothers include, for example, sexuality of the breasts. These factors combined with lack of self-efficacy and confidence mean that breastfeeding is experienced as stressful for young mothers (Poole & Gephart 2014) They also tend to report that interactions with healthcare providers are stressful, which suggests that interactions with health professionals may not be sufficiently woman-centred (MacVicar et al 2015).

A metasynthesis of 8 studies reporting on the support needs of young mothers and women from socially deprived backgrounds found that mothers from these groups want to receive a person-centred approach from health professionals who provide practical help to develop the skill of breastfeeding combined with psychological support (MacVicar et al 2015). This is not so different from the support needs of all women (Marshall et al 2007). However, sometimes midwives and others supporting mothers assume that young mothers and mothers from disadvantaged groups will formula feed and this, combined with difficulties they may have interacting with health professionals, can become a self-fulfilling prophecy.

It is essential that generalized and simplistic social and cultural descriptions are avoided. Midwives need to be aware that culture plays a role in women's breastfeeding experiences but to be sensitive to differences within various groups and similarities across groups. Crucially, midwives must actively listen to each woman to understand their individual needs and to appreciate that a woman's beliefs may not always match their own.

Activity

To provide culturally competent care, it is important that you understand your own personal reactions to cultural differences. When a person views the world from their own ethnic or cultural system, this is known as ethnocentrism, and this can be avoided by recognizing and appreciating cultural differences (Wambach 2016). Think of a woman you have cared for who held beliefs that were different from your own. Consider how you can show respect for her beliefs and how you can build on these in the infant feeding support you might provide.

REFLECTION ON THE TRIGGER SCENARIO

Sally has just arrived 'home' to her mother's house from the hospital with her partner Joe. They are staying with Sally's mother for a few weeks before moving into their own house. Sally had wanted to have her baby at home as she hated hospitals but had to be transferred to hospital during labour. After baby Eva was born, Sally was distraught because she did not have the opportunity to breastfeed within the first hour (she had read that this was important), but she enjoyed the 'special moment' when she finally breastfed. Sally breastfed Eva a couple of times but was then struggling and asked for help from the midwives. A range of different suggestions were offered by midwives who were very willing to help but seemed very busy. None of the suggestions seemed to help, and Sally had been left feeling confused and upset. Sally is now feeling much more relaxed at home with her mother as she is confident her mother can help if needed as she has breastfed all of her children. Sally's partner, Joe, is supportive emotionally but has already suggested Sally should give Eva a bottle of formula.

Sally felt uncomfortable in the hospital setting, but once at home, she felt much more relaxed. This scenario is based on a situation encountered in clinical practice as part of a research study (with all names changed). It demonstrates how support from family can help women to sustain breastfeeding but can also be rather mixed.

Sally explained how her mother helped her to continue to breastfeed at home. However, like many women, Sally felt her partner did not know how to help. She described him as supportive but said – 'he doesn't really know what to do, ... he's been an absolute star as far everything else, looking after the baby, as far as being awake all hours doing all the changes, looking after her, playing with her, taking her out and what have you, he's been fine, but I don't think he could do much as far as breastfeeding is concerned. I mean he sits there and he kind of puts his arms around me, in a sort of like there, there, I know your nipples hurt, poor you. He is kind of emotionally supportive, but he hasn't got the foggiest idea how to breastfeed or where to begin helping somebody to breastfeed, and I mean he was a lot more keen than me to just give her a bottle'. Sally also had a good relationship with her community midwife who she trusted implicitly.

How might the community midwife have involved Joe? Do you think it might have been helpful for him to attend antenatal education sessions? Do you think fathers and other family members always feel comfortable to attend? What more might be done to encourage this?

This scenario highlights how women's behaviour, choices and actions can be facilitated or constrained by the people around them. Now that you are familiar with issues relating to the social context of infant feeding, you should have insight into how the scenario relates to the evidence. The jigsaw model will now be used to explore the trigger scenario in more depth.

Effective communication

To provide appropriate infant feeding support to women, effective communication is essential. In particular, much can be gained from actively listening to women's experiences, beliefs and concerns. Questions that arise from the scenario might include: How might Sally have been better prepared for her experience of breastfeeding Eva? Might it have been helpful to involve Joe in conversations or sessions to prepare for parenthood and infant feeding? Sally was a young mother of 21 years old; might this mean she felt more or less able to ask for help whilst in the hospital? How might Sally's dislike of hospitals have impacted on her ability to communicate with the midwives caring for her? What questions might the midwife ask to encourage Sally to talk to find out about her current knowledge, understanding and beliefs about infant feeding?

Woman-centred care

It is clear that women want infant feeding support that is centred on their individual concerns and needs (MacVicar et al 2015) and that generalized non-specific information that could be given to anyone is not considered to be as helpful (Marshall et al 2007). A facilitative approach to support, within which skills are demonstrated and explanations given as to why a particular course of action might work, are more likely to be deemed helpful and empower women to resolve issues that might occur later. Questions that arise from the scenario might include: How might midwives in the hospital provide specific support for Sally? The community midwife had developed a strong relationship with Sally and this meant Sally trusted her implicitly; how will this have helped the midwife to provide effective infant feeding support? How do you ensure that support you provide for women meets their needs appropriately?

Using best evidence

Information provided by midwives to support mothers to feed their babies should be based on the most up-to-date available evidence, but this does not mean support should be routine or the same for all women. The midwife should find out what the woman knows already and build on this in a culturally sensitive, facilitative way. Questions that arise from the scenario might include: How might hospital midwives have done things differently to avoid Sally feeling like she was being provided with conflicting information? What information might the community midwife have given Joe when he was keen for Sally to give Eva a bottle feed? What would you say or do if a cultural practice does not fit with your understanding of current evidence and you felt it may compromise the health of the baby?

Professional and legal issues

To provide appropriate and effective care that meets the needs of individual women, midwives must practice in a way that responds to their concerns whilst also using the best available evidence (NMC 2015). The Code (NMC 2015) also requires midwives to act in the best interests of people at all times. In this scenario, questions that might be addressed include: Have the midwives supporting Sally and her family been trained at least to the minimum standards set out by the UNICEF Baby Friendly Initiative? What national guidelines provide evidence about infant feeding? Will these apply to all women? How would the community midwife document care and support she provided for Sally and Eva?

Team working

The midwife is responsible for providing infant feeding support to women in the early days after birth until the care of the women is transferred to the health visitor. Whether working in the hospital postnatal ward or the community setting, the midwife may work with other midwives, other health professionals, peer supporters and importantly with the woman's family. Questions that arise from the scenario might include: The infant feeding support provided for Sally in the hospital postnatal ward could have been more helpful to her as she left her feeling confused; how might this have been improved? How could the care provided to Sally and Eva have been communicated between members of the team on the postnatal ward? How and where should this care have been documented? What would have been helpful for the community midwife to know after Sally went home? Do you think Sally might have found peer support helpful?

Clinical dexterity

Women need to learn how to feed their baby quickly after their baby is born as it is life-giving to the baby. The skills a midwife needs to support women include effective communication skills that enable the provision of the right information at the right time and the technical skills required to enable women to position and attach their baby at the breast. Questions that arise from the scenario might include: How might the midwife demonstrate the skills of positioning and attachment? What visual aids might the midwife use to help Sally to understand the principles of how a baby feeds? How will the midwife ensure that she does this in a culturally sensitive way?

Models of care

Women receive care in a range of settings depending on the choices they make. Sometimes, as was the case for Sally, their wishes cannot be met due to circumstances outside their control. If Sally's wish to have a home birth had been possible, her early experiences of infant feeding might have been rather different. Questions that arise from the scenario might include: What factors might have been important to Sally if she had given birth at home and been attended by the community midwife who she knew and trusted? Might Joe have been able to be more involved in the early hours and days after birth? What effect might the perception that midwives are very busy have on Sally's ability to ask for help with breastfeeding on the postnatal ward? If the model of care Sally had received had been from a small team of midwives, would this have changed her experience? If so, how?

Safe environment

It is important the midwives ensure mothers and babies are in a safe environment whilst feeding. Parents should be made aware of the association between Sudden Infant Death Syndrome (SIDS) and falling asleep with their baby on a sofa. They should also be informed that the risk of co-sleeping may be greater if their baby is premature or parents have consumed alcohol or taken drugs. The safest place for the baby to sleep is in a cot in the same room (NICE 2006). Questions that arise from the scenario might include: Are Sally and Joe aware of the safe sleeping guidance? Might Sally or Joe fall asleep with Eva unintentionally? What advice would you give to Sally if you were the midwife on the postnatal ward? What advice would you give to Sally if you were the community midwife?

Promotes health

Evidence for the benefits of breastfeeding to the health of both mother and infant continue to accumulate (see, for example, Hoddinott et al 2008; Horta et al 2007; Victora et al 2016). Many women do understand that breastfeeding is 'best' for the baby; however, without skilled, sensitive support mothers who have chosen to start breastfeeding may not continue. Questions that arise from the scenario might include: What information about the benefits of breastfeeding should the midwife provide? How can this information be conveyed in a way that does not cause women to feel pressured? When should discussions about breastfeeding and health take place?

Further scenarios

The following scenarios enable you to consider how specific situations influence the care the midwife provides. Use the jigsaw model to explore the issues raised in each situation.

SCENARIO 1

The community midwife is talking to Paula during a postnatal visit. Paula's second baby, Emily, is now 10 days old, and she has been enjoying feeding her. She is concerned because they have just been away for the weekend to a family gathering, and Emily became unsettled, cried and needed feeding more often than usual. This led to comments of some of the older family members who said, 'Oh, you need to talk to your midwife or health visitor, because it doesn't look as if you've got enough milk there or it might not be strong enough'.

Practice point

Women often hear stories of friends or family who say they did not have enough milk or express concerns about the quality of it. Changes in the baby's behaviour can often undermine women's confidence in the light of these. Such exchanges can worry mothers and undermine their views of themselves as good mothers.

Further questions specific to Scenario 1 may be:
1. If you were the community midwife visiting Paula, how might you reassure her that she will produce enough breast milk?
2. What visible signs that Emily is getting enough milk could you discuss with Paula?
3. Would you observe Emily feeding?
4. How might you discuss responsive feeding and feeding cues?
5. Do you think Paula might benefit from talking to other breastfeeding mothers?
6. How might you encourage Paula to develop ways of dealing with comments that undermine breastfeeding from people in her social network?

Khaleda gave birth to her baby yesterday, and he has fed well at the breast after birth and since on the postnatal ward. Amy is a midwife working on the postnatal ward and is caring for Khaleda. She is surprised when Khaleda asks if her baby needs a bottle feed now.

Practice point

In the early days, many women need reassurance in relation to infant feeding. Some women simply want a midwife to observe their baby feeding to confirm that they are 'doing it right' (Marshall et al 2007:2153) whereas other women need more help and explanations. It is crucial to understand women's expectations in relation to postnatal care and infant feeding support as these may vary considerably. For example, McFadden et al (2012a) found that the expectation that women would return to normal activity immediately following birth was at odds with the situation in Bangladesh where women who have just given birth have 'special status' and receive intensive support to enable them to rest and nurture their baby. This same study highlights that, for women of Bangladeshi origin, it was struggling to establish breastfeeding and not receiving the support they expected combined with concern about the adequacy of breast milk that encouraged women to introduce formula feeds (McFadden et al 2012b). It was clear that some women would have liked more information as demonstrated in this quote: *'I want to ask this thing that at that time there is no milk, during the first few days, 2, 3 days after the birth there is no milk so why do they keep on telling me to get them to suck and feed'* (McFadden et al 2012a:128).

Further questions specific to Scenario 2 include:
1. If you were the midwife on the postnatal ward caring for Khaleda, how might you have responded?
2. If Khaleda does not understand and speak English, what interpreter services are available in your area?
3. What open question might you ask?
4. How would you ensure that your response is culturally sensitive?
5. What could you explain to Khaleda about the amount and composition of colostrum?
6. How might you involve family members?

Conclusion

It is essential for midwives to try to find out and to understand the social context within which breastfeeding occurs for each woman in her care. Although it has been known for some time that extra support improves breastfeeding outcomes, women still do not always feel well supported. Midwives have an important role to play in both supporting women with technical and emotional aspects of breastfeeding in the early days and helping women to mobilize other forms of support such as group-based peer support and/or family or informal social support later on.

References

Barlow, J., Coe, C., Redshaw, M., Underdown, A., 2009. Birth and Beyond: Stakeholder Perceptions of Current Antenatal Education Provision in England. Warwick Infant and Family Wellbeing Unit, University of Warwick, National Perinatal Epidemiology Unit, Oxford.

Dykes, F., 2006. Breastfeeding in Hospital: Mothers, Midwives and the Production Line. Routledge, Abingdon.

Häggkvist, A.-P., Brantsæter, A.L., Grjibovski, A.M., et al., 2010. Prevalence of breast-feeding in the Norwegian Mother and Child Cohort Study and health service-related correlates of cessation of full breast-feeding. Public Health Nutr. 13, 2076–2086.

Hoddinott, P., Chalmers, M., Pill, R., 2006. One-to-one or group-based peer support for breastfeeding? Women's perceptions of a breastfeeding peer coaching intervention. Birth 33, 139–146.

Hoddinott, P., Craig, L.C.A., Britten, J., McInnes, R.M., 2012. A serial qualitative interview study of infant feeding experiences: idealism meets realism. BMJ Open 2 (2), e000504. doi:10.1136/bmjopen-2011-000504.

Hoddinott, P., Pill, R., 1999. Qualitative study of decisions about infant feeding among women in east end of London. BMJ 318, 30–34.

Hoddinott, P., Tappin, D., Wright, C., 2008. Breast feeding. BMJ 336, 881–887.

Horta, B.L., Bahl, R., Martines, J.C., Victora, C.G., 2007. Evidence on the Long-Term Effects of Breastfeeding: Systematic Reviews and Meta-Analyses. World Health Organization, Geneva.

MacVicar, S., Kirkpatrick, P., Humphrey, T., Forbes-McKay, K.E., 2015. Supporting breastfeeding establishment among socially disadvantaged women: a meta-synthesis. Birth 42, 290–298.

Marshall, J., Godfrey, M., 2012. Shifting identities: social and cultural factors that shape decision-making around breastfeeding. In: Liamputtong, P. (Ed.), Infant Feeding Practices: A Cross Cultural Perspective. Springer, New York.

Marshall, J.L., Godfrey, M., Renfrew, M.J., 2007. Being a 'good mother': managing breastfeeding and merging identities. Soc. Sci. Med. 65, 2147–2159.

McAndrew, F., Thompson, J., Fellows, L., et al., 2012. Infant Feeding Survey 2010. Health and Social Care Information Centre, London.

McFadden, A., Gavine, A., Renfrew, M.J., et al., 2017. Support for healthy breastfeeding mothers with healthy term babies. Cochrane Database Syst. Rev. (2), Art. No.: CD001141, doi:10.1002/14651858.CD001141.pub5.

McFadden, A., Renfrew, M.J., Atkin, K., 2012a. Does cultural context make a difference to women's experiences of maternity care? A qualitative study comparing the perspectives of breast-feeding women of Bangladeshi origin and health practitioners. Health Expect. 16, e124.

McFadden, A., Renfrew, M.J., Atkin, K., 2012b. Using qualitative research findings to analyse how breastfeeding public health recommendations can be tailored to meet the needs of women of Bangladeshi origin living in England. J. Res. Nurs. 17, 159–178.

Murphy, E., 1999. 'Breast is best': Infant feeding decisions and maternal deviance. Sociol. Health Illn. 21, 187–208.

NICE, 2006. Routine Postnatal Care of Women and Their Babies. NICE, London.

NMC, 2015. The Code: Professional Standards of Practice and Behaviour for Nurses and Midwives. Nursing and Midwifery Council., London. Available at:: https://www.nmc.org.uk/globalassets/sitedocuments/nmc-publications/nmc-code.pdf.

Poole, S.N., Gephart, S.M., 2014. State of the science for practice to promote breastfeeding success among young mothers. Newborn Infant Nurs. Rev. 14, 112.

Schmied, V., Beake, S., Sheehan, A., et al., 2011. Women's perceptions and experiences of breastfeeding support: a metasynthesis. Birth 38, 49–60.

Victora, C.G., Bahl, R., Barros, A.J.D., et al., 2016. Breastfeeding in the 21st century: epidemiology, mechanisms, and lifelong effect. Lancet 387, 475–490.

Wambach, K., 2016. The cultural context of breastfeeding. In: Wambach, K., Riordan, J. (Eds.), Breastfeeding and Human Lactation. Jones and Bartlett, Burlington.

CHAPTER 7

Birthing practices and breastfeeding

TRIGGER SCENARIO

Alison is pregnant for the first time, and she has chosen to have her baby in the local hospital. She is in labour and being supported by her partner, Jim, and Steph, who is a doula. Alison has been coping with the pain of labour very well so far; she has been mobile throughout the early stages, she has been using a birthing ball and Jim has been massaging her back. Alison has just told Kelly, the midwife caring for her in labour, 'I need an epidural now'.

Introduction

Supporting normal birth in environments where mothers feel relaxed results in shorter, easier births which means mothers and babies are likely to be healthier and more alert as they start their breastfeeding journey (Smith & Kroeger 2010). Conversely, babies exposed to long and difficult labours and/or assisted birth often have difficulty feeding. Although there are gaps in the research evidence, many links have been investigated. Not all situations that have the potential to affect feeding can be changed as they are necessary to protect the health of the mother and baby, but minimizing unnecessary interventions and providing a relaxed and supportive labour environment is essential.

The effects of these labour practices can be minimized by good care after birth. A baby who has unhurried and uninterrupted skin-to-skin contact with their mother immediately after birth is much more likely to crawl to the breast and suckle even if 'sleepy' from medication given during labour (Righard & Alade 1990). Babies who are separated from their mothers are less likely to suckle, are more stressed by birth and cry more, increasing the risk of post-birth intracranial bleeds (Genna 2013). Therefore for these reasons, as well as enhancing the relationship between the mother and baby (see Chapters 2 and 3), mothers should be encouraged to spend as much time as possible in skin-to-skin contact with their baby and to recognize feeding cues. Further management of feeding difficulties occurring as a result of situations during labour or birth injuries will vary depending on the condition. Obtaining a good labour history is therefore important if a baby is reluctant to feed after birth.

UNICEF Baby Friendly Maternity standards

The following are the maternity standards that are most relevant to this chapter:

- Support all mothers and babies to initiate a close relationship and feeding soon after birth
- Enable mothers to get breastfeeding off to a good start

UNICEF Baby Friendly UK University learning outcomes

The following are the learning outcomes that are achieved within this chapter. By the end of their midwifery education programme, students will:

- Have sufficient knowledge of anatomy of the breast and physiology of lactation to enable them to support mothers to successfully establish and maintain breastfeeding
- Be able to apply their knowledge and understanding of the physiology of lactation to support women to get breastfeeding off to a good start
- Have the knowledge and skills to access the evidence that underpins infant feeding practice

---

Support during labour

Historically, women tended to be supported by other women during labour and birth. However, the move to the majority of women birthing in a hospital during the 1960s and 1970s has led to this no longer being common practice. If women feel relaxed and empowered during birth, they are likely to labour more easily and to receive fewer interventions, and this is more likely if women are well supported. Women in labour are particularly sensitive to the environment and, in the hospital, they are often subjected to factors such as routines, high levels of intervention and lack of privacy that may impact on their labour and birth, and this ultimately has the potential to affect their transition to motherhood and breastfeeding experiences.

Labour support might include aspects such as reassurance, praise and other emotional support combined with providing comfort, such as touch, massage and food and drink. Information about coping techniques and labour progress may also be needed along with advocacy to enable the women to express their wishes. A Cochrane review of 22 trials involving 15,288 women has investigated the effect of one-to-one care in labour in a range of settings (Hodnett et al 2013). The findings show that when women receive continuous support care in labour, their labours tend to be slightly shorter, women are less likely to need analgesia and they are more likely to have spontaneous vaginal births. It has been postulated that these factors might lead to improved breastfeeding outcomes. However, within this Cochrane review, there were only three trials that reported on breastfeeding as an outcome, and the review did not find an association between support in labour and breastfeeding 1 to 2 months after birth (Hodnett et al 2013).

This does not necessarily mean that providing support during labour does not have any effect on breastfeeding because the evidence from this review that can throw light on this link is not strong. For example, if all trials included had assessed breastfeeding as an outcome, an association may have been apparent, or perhaps breastfeeding is affected initially, but extra support for women has the potential to resolve the issues by 2 months. Ultimately, the labour environment and the support women receive during labour can impact on other factors such as length of labour and whether or not and when pharmacological pain relief is needed. It is essential to understand that the drugs that are often given in labour may affect the mother and baby and therefore have potential to impact on breastfeeding. An overview of the effects of the main labour and birth interventions on breastfeeding is provided (Table 7.1).

Drugs routinely given in labour and breastfeeding

Women in labour experience pain differently and have a range of ways of coping with it. Women may use a variety of strategies to help, such as emersion in water, acupuncture, relaxation techniques and massage. A recent overview of Cochrane reviews has suggested that although, due to lack of studies the efficacy of such non-pharmacological methods is unclear these methods may help women to manage labour pain and appear to be safe for mother and baby (Jones et al 2012). However, many women do wish to have pain-relieving drugs during labour whether or not they have used other ways of coping.

Different types of drugs given in labour affect the mother and the baby in a range of ways. They may affect the baby's ability to feed, the mother's willingness or ability to let her baby feed or the physiological production of breastmilk. In the following sections, both the mechanisms through which the various drugs might affect breastfeeding and current best evidence will be discussed. However, there is a paucity of high-quality studies demonstrating clear links between methods of pain relief in labour and breastfeeding.

Table 7.1: Labour and birth interventions and likely effect on the baby

Labour and birth interventions	Likely effects on the baby
Induction of labour	• Prostaglandins are dopamine agonists which are known to suppress prolactin secretion • May interfere with endogenous patterns of oxytocin secretion and sensitivity of oxytocin receptors • Infant is more likely to be immature
Opioids during labour	• Depress respiratory function – linked to inability to coordinate sucking, swallowing and breathing • Make the baby sleepy and unresponsive and can delay effective feeding • Effects are dose related
Epidural anaesthesia	• All drugs used in epidurals reach the fetus in varying amounts within 10 minutes so may have a direct effect • Indirect effects include factors such as women remaining supine which slows progress of labour, reduces the baby's ability to cope with pain through lack of beta-endorphines in colostrum
Caesarean birth	• Caesarean birth may interfere with the natural production and release of hormones. Women who have had caesarean births have fewer oxytocin pulses in relation to breastfeeding 2–3 days after birth when compared with women who have had a vaginal birth
Long labour and assisted birth, either forceps or ventouse extraction	• Can cause cranial asymmetry of the occipital bones that can contribute to poor suck
Suctioning to posterior oropharynx	• Babies may have resulting oral aversions making breastfeeding difficult
Uterotonics for third stage	• Have been associated with lower rates of breastfeeding

Sources (Jordan et al 2005; Smith 2013, Smith & Kroeger 2010, Uvnas-Moberg 2011; Walker 2017).

Opioids and breastfeeding

Opioids cross the placenta to the fetus by diffusion and can cause respiratory depression. It has been estimated that if, for example, the mother has been given Pethidine during labour, it may take the baby 3 to 6 days to process and eliminate this from his system (Jones et al 2012). Although most of the drug may be metabolized within 2 or 3 days (Hogg et al 1977), the amount in the baby's system will be affected by the interval between administration of the drug and birth. Observational studies have shown that if mothers have had opioids during labour, after birth the baby is less alert and does not display breast-seeking behaviours in the same ways as babies of un-medicated mothers, resulting in delayed breastfeeding (Ransjö-Arvidson et al 2001; Righard & Alade 1990). Suckling may also be affected, and babies of medicated mothers tend to lose the ability to breath, suck and swallow in a coordinated way.

Although the use of opioids is common and there has been concern about their effects on babies for at least 30 years, there is little evidence from randomized controlled trials of the effects of opioids on the ability of the baby to suckle and to initiate breastfeeding (Ullman et al 2010). Despite this lack of evidence from randomized controlled trials, it is clear from observational studies that the baby's ability to initiate breastfeeding is affected when the mother has had opioids in labour. If the baby is not able to initiate breastfeeding or does not feed well, this can eventually result in milk stasis and affect milk production. However, it is less clear whether this has a lasting impact on breastfeeding. Early studies suggest that the effects can be reduced by ensuring that baby has immediate, unhurried skin-to-skin contact with the mother (Righard & Alade 1990).

Activity

When you next work within a birth environment, observe the baby's behaviour immediately after birth and the first feed. Do you notice any difference in the behaviour of babies whose mothers have had opioids during labour?

Epidural and breastfeeding

Epidural anaesthesia provides effective pain relief for women in labour (Anim-Somuah et al 2011); however, a recent systematic review investigating the association between epidural anaesthesia and breastfeeding outcome was inconclusive (French et al 2016). This review identified relevant studies from a range of different countries, including the UK, and in 12 studies, epidural anaesthesia was associated with lower breastfeeding rates. But in a further 10 studies, there was no association, and in one study, there appeared to be a positive association (French et al 2016). This variation might be explained by issues, such as the size and/or lack of quality in some of the studies, including that some do not measure or take account of factors that are known to be associated with breastfeeding, such as breastfeeding intention.

It is difficult to conclusively ascertain cause and effect associations between one labour intervention and breastfeeding. Labour interventions often occur in a cascade and are therefore linked. For example, epidural anaesthesia in labour leads to an increased chance of longer second stage and augmentation with oxytocin (Anim-Somuah et al 2011), so it is not necessarily possible to be sure whether it is the epidural or these other factors that affects breastfeeding.

The mechanisms by which epidural may impact on breastfeeding include direct effects of the drugs used on the baby and indirect effects such as encouraging a supine position during labour, which can lead to longer labour (Smith & Kroeger 2010). It is also thought that epidural may lead to lowering of oxytocin levels during and after birth (Uvnas-Moberg 2011). This may lead to reduced interactions between mother and baby and consequently delayed or poor initial breastfeeding (Rahm et al 2002). A baby sleepy from birth medications can be affected for several days, so expressed colostrum may need to be given by cup or syringe.

Activity

Consider how you might provide information to women about the effect of different methods of pain relief on breastfeeding. When would be the most appropriate time to do this in your place of work? Are there other midwives or health professionals you might involve in discussions about this?

Uterotonics and breastfeeding

Uterotonics such as oxytocin and prostaglandin that are used for induction and augmentation of labour may also affect breastfeeding. Prostaglandins administered for induction of labour have been shown in a UK cohort study to be associated with lower breastfeeding rates 48 hours after birth (Jordan et al 2005). This may be because prostaglandins are dopamine agonists which are known to suppress prolactin secretion (Jordan et al 2005). Synthetic oxytocin used for induction of labour may interfere with natural patterns of oxytocin release during labour and affect the sensitivity of oxytocin receptors. In addition to these possible mechanisms, when labour is induced, contractions are likely to be more painful and closer together, and this is therefore associated with increased use of opioids and epidural for pain relief, and the mother and baby may be affected as previously discussed.

Interestingly, Jordan et al (2005) also found that, in the group of women having their first baby who had received nitrous oxide, breastfeeding rates were higher. They suggest that this finding might be explained by the link between stress and impaired natural oxytocin release that might be reduced in women receiving nitrous oxide. However, this protective effect was only seen in women having their first baby; when all women were included, the association was not apparent (Jordan et al 2005).

This same large cohort study that was conducted in Wales also found associations between administration of uterotonics for the prevention of postpartum haemorrhage (PPH) and reduced breastfeeding rates. This included oxytocin alone or combined with ergometrine by all routes of administration, and rates of breastfeeding appeared to be reduced by 6% to 8% (Jordan et al 2005). The routine use of uterotonics as part of active management of the third stage of labour aims to reduce postpartum haemorrhage (PPH), and the use of oxytocin is recommended by National Institute for Health and Care Excellence (NICE 2014). However, it may be that some women may prefer to choose to avoid the use of uterotonics if they knew of the possible association with reduced breastfeeding rates.

Activity

'Oxytocin is both a hormone, which acts in the body through the blood stream, and a signalling substance in the nervous system' (Uvnas-Moberg 2011:61). Read about the physiology of oxytocin and consider how this might be affected by giving synthetic oxytocin. Consider the possible link between active management of labour and reduced breastfeeding rates and the possible increased risk of PPH. How might you explain this to women to enable them to make an informed choice about the third stage of labour?

Caesarean section and breastfeeding

A recent cohort study conducted in Canada found that when women have had a planned caesarean birth, their babies are less likely to be breastfeeding when they are 12 weeks old (Hobbs et al 2016). This study also found that women who have had their baby by caesarean birth are more likely to experience breastfeeding difficulties initially (Hobbs et al 2016), which reinforces the findings of a large international meta-analysis of 53 studies

(Prior et al 2012). This study also found that, overall, babies born by caesarean were less likely to be breastfed at 6 months of age; however, if breastfeeding was initiated, there was no difference in rates at 6 months (Prior et al 2012).

This therefore suggests that women who have had a caesarean birth are more likely to need support to initiate breastfeeding. A small qualitative study of eight women's experiences of breastfeeding after caesarean section carried out in Australia highlights that these women felt helpless and tired after birth, they were disappointed not to be able to have skin-to-skin contact with their baby in theatre and they did not feel able to care for their baby in the first 24 hours after birth (Chaplin et al 2016). These mothers also described their babies' tiredness and inability to suck, explained that they received conflicting information from midwives, that they were concerned they did not have enough milk and that all of this left them feeling disappointed, frustrated and with a sense of failure (Chaplin et al 2016).

Caesarean birth may interfere with the natural production and release of hormones for both mother and baby. Women who have had caesarean births have fewer oxytocin pulses in relation to breastfeeding 2 to 3 days after birth when compared with women who have had a vaginal birth (Uvnas-Moberg 2011). The cause of these differences could be due to reduced release of oxytocin during birth or alternatively might be related to delayed skin-to-skin contact or pain and stress of the surgery. When a mother does not labour, such as when she has an elective caesarean birth, fetal endorphins are reduced as are endorphins present in the colostrum and breastmilk, resulting in less pain relief for the baby (Smith & Kroeger 2010).

Activity

Skin-to-skin contact is beneficial for all women but may be particularly helpful to women who have had caesarean birth. Is skin-to-skin contact between mother and baby in theatre common practice in your area? How might you encourage this practice? Consider the different professionals you might need to involve in any discussions to encourage this practice.

Trauma to the baby at birth

Babies can sometimes have trauma to their face and head following birth. After a spontaneous vaginal birth, caput succedaneum and moulding of the baby's skull bones are commonly seen. However, if the baby has been born by forceps or vacuum extraction, they may have further bruising on their face or even occasionally lacerations. Such injuries may simply cause pain meaning that the baby may be reluctant to suck, but in a few babies a condition known as Torticollis (Latin for *twisted neck*) has been described. Wall and Glass (2006) reported on 11 case studies of infants with this condition and suggest that it is linked to impaired sucking in newborn babies.

If a mother has been in labour, fetal endorphins will be present both in the baby and in the breastmilk, which will help to alleviate any pain following birth. If a baby has trauma from an instrumental birth, a feeding position, such as laid-back breastfeeding where the baby's head is not touched, may be most successful as this will illicit the baby's reflexes and the mother's nurturing instincts (Colson 2005); a quiet and calm environment may also be helpful. A careful examination for asymmetry at this early stage may also enable the midwife to identify any problems and lead to closer observation of the baby's ability to suck and milk transfer.

REFLECTION ON THE TRIGGER SCENARIO

Look back at the trigger scenario.

> Alison is pregnant for the first time, and she has chosen to have her baby in the local hospital. She is in labour and being supported by her partner, Jim, and Steph, who is a doula. Alison has been coping with the pain of labour very well so far; she has been mobile throughout the early stages, she has been using a birthing ball and Jim has been massaging her back. Alison has just told Kelly, the midwife caring for her in labour, 'I need an epidural now'.

Alison may be approaching transition to the second stage of labour and with support may be able to continue to cope with the pain of labour. Kelly knows from previous conversations that Alison is very keen to breastfeed her baby. What information about the effect of epidural anaesthesia on breastfeeding might have been given to Alison? When might discussions about this be most appropriate?

This scenario highlights the difficulty of having in-depth discussions with women during labour. Now that you are familiar with some of the ways that common birthing practices might affect breastfeeding, you should have insight into how the scenario relates to the evidence. The jigsaw model will now be used to explore the trigger scenario in more depth.

Effective communication

Communicating the concept of risk to women is not always straightforward. Many of these possible effects of labour interventions are not clearly linked to breastfeeding outcomes and many women will choose, for example, to have epidural anaesthesia. Therefore skilful and sensitive communication is needed to ensure that women understand the possible risks but in a way that does not mean they feel they have 'failed' if they do want some form of analgesia during labour. Questions that arise from the scenario might include: Did the midwife discuss types of pain relief available in labour with Alison during antenatal appointments? Did Alison and Jim attend preparation for parenting sessions? Did this information build on their existing knowledge and understanding? What had Alison recorded in her birth plan?

Woman-centred care

Types of pain relief that are available to women during labour are discussed during the antenatal period, either during preparation for parenting sessions or through discussions within antenatal appointments. However, links between the different methods of pain relief and breastfeeding are less often discussed. To provide women-centred care, women must be enabled to make choices and therefore should be provided with information about this. Questions that arise from the scenario might include: What does Alison understand about the possible effects of epidural anaesthesia on herself and the baby and ultimately breastfeeding? When do you think these discussions might have occurred? How might Jim have been involved? What role might Alison's doula, Steph, have?

Using best evidence

Although there have been a number of relevant Cochrane reviews on labour interventions, many of the trials included in these have not assessed breastfeeding as an outcome. This means that there is not strong evidence for some of the links discussed in this chapter. However, it is important to continue to question the effects of routine labour interventions and to understand the physiology and mechanisms that may underpin any possible negative effects on breastfeeding. Questions that might arise from the scenario include: Do Alison and Jim understand the possible effects of epidural anaesthesia? Might there be other options to help Alison cope with the pain of labour? If you were the midwife explaining the possible effects of different types of pain relief in labour, what would you say to Alison and Jim?

Professional and legal issues

Midwives must practice safely and protect women and babies from potential harm (NMC 2015). Midwives will therefore need to consider how what happens during labour may affect the health and wellbeing of the mother and baby after birth. For example, this may include providing information to women about the effects of the different types of pain relief on the baby to enable her to make an informed choice. In this scenario, questions that may be asked include: Are there local or national guidelines that relate to pain relief and other interventions in labour? To what extent are these guidelines evidence-based? When might the various interventions, such as pain relief, that the woman may request during labour be discussed in detail? Would it be helpful if Jim was involved in these discussions? How would the midwife document discussions with Alison and Jim about options for care in labour and possible adverse effects of these?

Team working

Although the midwife is responsible for the care of the mother during labour and birth, it is important that she works with others. In this scenario, this would include Alison's partner, Jim, and her doula, Steph. She may also need to liaise with other midwives and members of the medical team, for example, an anaesthetist for siting an epidural or a doctor should any complications occur. Questions that arise from the scenario might include: How might the midwife work with Alison's doula, Steph, to ensure optimal support? How might she ensure that Jim's needs are also met so that he can also support Alison? How would the midwife document care in labour so that midwives on the postnatal ward have all the information they might need to continue to provide seamless care?

Clinical dexterity

The midwife supporting a woman before and during birth needs to have a comprehensive understanding of the current evidence relating to interventions during labour, and this should include possible effects on breastfeeding. Many clinical skills are required when caring for women in labour, but sensitive communication and empathetic support are essential. Questions that arise from the scenario might include: What do women expect from the midwife providing care in labour? How might Kelly increase Alison's ability to cope with pain in labour? What further options might Kelly suggest?

Models of care

Women who receive midwifery-led continuity models of care are more likely to have a spontaneous vaginal birth and less likely to have an epidural, instrumental vaginal birth or experience fetal loss (Sandall et al 2016). Women who experience midwifery-led models of care are also more likely to be cared for in labour by a midwife they know (Sandall et al 2016). Questions that arise from the scenario might include: What model of care has Alison experienced? Does she have a named midwife caring for her? How might a midwife-led continuity model of care have enabled more comprehensive discussion about options for labour?

Safe environment

The midwife needs to ensure that she provides a safe environment that is relaxing as possible for labouring women in her care. When a woman feels more relaxed in labour this will enhance production of hormones such as oxytocin, ultimately leading to a higher likelihood of a spontaneous vaginal birth. Questions that arise from the scenario might include: Is there anything the midwife can do to the environment to make it more relaxing for Alison? What strategies might she suggest for Alison? Is the bed in the middle of the labour room? If so, might it be more helpful to one side of the room against a wall?

Promotes health

Ensuring continuous support for women in labour is likely to mean a woman will have a shorter labour and be less likely to need pain relief (Hodnett et al 2013). Ultimately, anything that reduces the need for interventions during labour is likely to lead to a higher chance that the baby will be able to breastfeed with fewer problems. Questions that might arise from the scenario include: What non-pharmacological interventions might have been suggested for Alison to help her to cope with pain during labour? Did the midwife discuss the possible side effects related to the use of uterotonics for the third stage of labour?

Further scenarios

The following scenarios enable you to consider how specific situations influence the care the midwife provides. Use the jigsaw model to explore the issues raised in each situation.

SCENARIO 1

Julia has chosen to breastfeed her baby. She had her baby, Joshua, by caesarean section yesterday and is now on the postnatal ward. She does not yet feel able to care for her baby because she is experiencing pain and is not yet very mobile.

Practice point

Mothers whose babies are born by caesarean section are less likely to start to breastfeed (Prior et al 2012). They may therefore need more support than other mothers to initiate breastfeeding. The reasons for this are likely to be multifactorial and include factors such as exposure to anaesthetic drugs; reduced exposure to oxytocin as a result of not going through labour and being less likely to have uninterrupted time skin-to-skin after birth in theatre.

Further points specific to Scenario 1 include:

1. How might the midwife caring for Julia use this opportunity to support her and her baby to have time in skin-to-skin contact together?
2. How might the midwife support Julia to breastfeed?
3. What might the midwife explain to Julia about the possible effects of the caesarean on the baby and breastfeeding?
4. What position might Julia find most comfortable to breastfeed her baby to avoid pain from the caesarean?
5. How might the midwife explain how a baby takes the breast to ensure Julia understands?

SCENARIO 2

Gillian is at the antenatal clinic talking to the midwife Valerie about her birth plan. Gillian has concerns about having medication for an active third stage of labour and has asked Valerie if there might be any advantages or disadvantages to deciding to have a physiological third stage of labour.

Practice point

Mothers should be encouraged to write a birth plan, but to make choices about birth they need balanced evidence-based information.

Further points specific to Scenario 2 include:

1. Why is syntocinon recommended by NICE (2006) for the third stage of labour?
2. What advantages of having an active third stage of labour might Valerie discuss with Gillian?
3. What disadvantages of having an active third stage of labour might Valerie discuss with Gillian?
4. What evidence might Valerie draw upon during this discussion?
5. Gillian is very keen to breastfeed her baby. What might Valerie explain about the link between active management of third stage of labour and breastfeeding?

Conclusion

The evidence for the effect of the various birthing practices on breastfeeding is accumulating but is still far from clear. However, the cascade of labour interventions that often occur is likely to work against the initiation of breastfeeding and the establishment of exclusive breastfeeding. These interventions may be reduced by practices such as one-to-one support during labour, and if they occur the effect on breastfeeding may be reduced by encouraging skin-to-skin contact and provision of skilled and sensitive support.

Resources

Cochrane Library. A range of reviews relating to the link between labour interventions and breastfeeding. Available at: http://www.cochranelibrary.com/.

Jones L, Othman M, Dowswell T, Alfirevic Z, Gates S, Newburn M, Jordan S, Lavender T & Neilson JP, 2012. Pain management for women in labour: an overview of systematic reviews. *The Cochrane Database of Systematic Reviews* Issue 3. Art. No.: CD00 9234. DOI:10.1002/14651858.CD009234.pub2.

National Institute for Health and Care Excellence, 2015. Postnatal care up to 8 weeks after birth. *Clinical Guideline 37*. London: National Collaborating Centre for Primary Care. Available at: https://www.nice.org.uk/guidance/cg37/resources/postnatal-care-up-to-8-weeks-after-birth-975391596997.

Smith LJ & Kroeger M, 2010. *Impact of birthing practices on breastfeeding*. London: Jones and Bartlett.

References

Anim-Somuah, M., Smyth, R.M.D., Jones, L., 2011. Epidural versus non-epidural or no analgesia in labour. Cochrane Database Syst. Rev. (12), CD000331. doi:10.1002/14651858.CD000331.pub3.

Chaplin, J., Kelly, J., Kildea, S., 2016. Maternal perceptions of breastfeeding difficulty after caesarean section with regional anaesthesia: A qualitative study. Women Birth 29, 144–152.

Colson, S., 2005. Maternal breastfeeding positions: have we got it right? (2). Pract. Midwife 8, 29–32.

French, C.A., Cong, X., Chung, K.S., 2016. Labor epidural analgesia and breastfeeding: a systematic review. J. Hum. Lact. 32, 507–520.

Genna, C.W., 2013. The influence of anatomic and structural issues on sucking skills. In: Genna, C.W. (Ed.), Supporting Suckling Skills in Breastfeeding Infants, second ed. Jones and Bartlett, New York.

Hobbs, A.J., Mannion, C.A., McDonald, S.W., et al., 2016. The impact of caesarean section on breastfeeding initiation, duration and difficulties in the first four months postpartum. BMC Pregnancy Childbirth 16, 90.

Hodnett, E.D., Gates, S., Hofmeyr, G.J., Sakala, C., 2013. Continuous support for women during childbirth. Cochrane Database Syst. Rev. (7), CD003766. doi:10.1002/14651858.CD003766.pub5.

Hogg, M.I., Wiener, P.C., Rosen, M., Mapleson, W.W., 1977. Urinary excretion and metabolism of pethidine and norpethidine in the newborn. Br. J. Anaesth. 49, 891–899.

Jones, L., Othman, M., Dowswell, T., et al., 2012. Pain management for women in labour: an overview of systematic reviews. Cochrane Database Syst. Rev. (3), CD009234. doi:10.1002/14651858.CD009234.pub2.

Jordan, S., Emery, S., Bradshaw, C., et al., 2005. The impact of intrapartum analgesia on infant feeding. BJOG 112, 927–934.

National Institute for Health and Care Excellence, 2014. Intrapartum care: care for healthy women and babies. NICE CG190. Available at: https://www.nice.org.uk/guidance/cg190. (Accessed 8 October 2016).

NICE, 2006. Routine Postnatal Care of Women and Their Babies. NICE, London.

NMC, 2015. The code: professional standards of practice and behaviour for nurses and midwives. London: Nursing and Midwifery Council. Available at: https://www.nmc.org.uk/globalassets/sitedocuments/nmc-publications/nmc-code.pdf.

Prior, E., Santhakumaran, S., Gale, C., et al., 2012. Breastfeeding after cesarean delivery: a systematic review and meta-analysis of world literature. Am. J. Clin. Nutr. 95, 1113–1135.

Rahm, V.-A., Hallgren, A., Högberg, H., et al., 2002. Plasma oxytocin levels in women during labor with or without epidural analgesia: a prospective study. Acta Obstet. Gynecol. Scand. 81, 1033–1039.

Ransjö-Arvidson, A., Matthiesen, A., Lilja, G., et al., 2001. Maternal analgesia during labor disturbs newborn behavior: effects on breastfeeding, temperature, and crying … including commentary by Kennell JH and McGrath S. Birth 28, 5.

Righard, L., Alade, M.O., 1990. Effect of delivery room routines on success of first breast-feed. Lancet 336, 1105–1107.

Sandall, J., Soltani, H., Gates, S., et al., 2016. Midwife-led continuity models versus other models of care for childbearing women. Cochrane Database Syst. Rev. (4), CD004667. doi:10.1002/14651858.CD004667.pub5.

Smith, L.J., 2013. Why Johnny can't suck: impact of birth practices on infant suck. In: Genna, C.W. (Ed.), Supporting Sucking Skills. Jones and Bartlett, London.

Smith, L.J., Kroeger, M., 2010. Impact of Birthing Practices on Breastfeeding. Jones and Bartlett, London.

Ullman, R., Smith, L., Burns, E., et al., 2010. Parenteral opioids for maternal pain management in labour. Cochrane Database Syst. Rev. (9), CD007396. doi:10.1002/14651858.CD007396.pub2.

Uvnas-Moberg, K., 2011. The Oxytocin Factor: Tapping the Hormone of Calm, Love and Healing. Pinter and Martin, London.

Walker, M., 2017. Breastfeeding Management for the Clinician: Using the Evidence, fourth ed. Jones and Bartlett, Burlington.

Wall, V., Glass, R., 2006. Mandibular asymmetry and breastfeeding problems: experience from 11 cases. J. Hum. Lact. 22, 328–334.

CHAPTER 8

Managing baby-related feeding challenges

TRIGGER SCENARIO

Laura was born during the night and is now lying on her mother's chest. She has started to stir and is beginning to move her head from side-to-side. Her mother, Bethany, looks down at her and smiles. Laura has been very sleepy since birth and only made a few attempts to suckle despite lying against her mother skin-to-skin most of the time since her birth. 'Come on Laura,' she said, 'you must be hungry now.'

Introduction

Whilst many babies will breastfeed soon after birth, this is not always the case. Many women and their babies encounter problems or challenges in the early days after birth, and this can lead to women choosing not to continue breastfeeding. In the UK, around 81% of women start to breastfeed, but by the time the baby is 1 week old, only 69% are still feeding, and by 6 weeks, this has fallen to 55% (McAndrew et al 2012). In the 2010 infant feeding survey, the reasons women gave for giving up breastfeeding in the first week after birth included: the baby not sucking or refusing the breast, painful breasts or nipples or that mothers felt they did not have enough milk (McAndrew et al 2012). Most women who took part in this survey wanted to breastfeed their baby for longer and felt that more support would have helped them to do so.

Some of the common initial challenges, such as a baby being reluctant to breastfeed, can be caused by a lack of understanding of the innate behaviours of the newborn baby and the environmental triggers for these (Genna & Sandora 2013). Interference with the normal sequence of the baby's breast-seeking behaviours (discussed in Chapter 4) may be responsible for some of these challenges and can usually be avoided by ensuring mothers and their newborn babies are enabled to have uninterrupted time in skin-to-skin contact after birth.

Many of the early challenges can be resolved with sensitive, unhurried support. High-quality sensitive support is appreciated by mothers and can help them to continue to breastfeed (McAndrew et al 2012). A breastfeeding mother appreciates the supporter observing the baby feed to provide reassurance that feeding is going well. Practical help to position and attach the baby (as discussed in Chapter 5) can resolve or prevent many issues that may arise. Sometimes if a baby is reluctant to feed biological nurturing, feeding in a laid-back position with the baby in close contact, can help as gravity elicits the baby's primitive reflexes and can enable both mother and baby to relax (Colson et al 2008). This can be particularly useful if a baby is pulling away from the breast or has trauma to the back of their head (see Chapter 7).

Babies may have congenital conditions that can mean that breastfeeding is a challenge, such as tongue-tie (Ankyloglossa) or cleft lip and palate. To appreciate the effect of such structural abnormalities, it is important to understand the normal mechanism of feeding (see Chapter 3). Babies may also develop conditions such as hypoglycaemia or jaundice early after birth that can impact on a baby's ability to breastfeed. This chapter outlines the basic knowledge required by the midwife caring for mothers and babies when such challenges occur.

UNICEF Baby Friendly Maternity standards

The following are the maternity standards that are most relevant to this chapter:
- Support all mothers and babies to initiate a close relationship and feeding soon after birth
- Enable mothers to get breastfeeding off to a good start

UNICEF Baby Friendly UK University learning outcomes

The following are the learning outcomes that are achieved within this chapter. By the end of their midwifery education programme, students will:
- Be able to apply their knowledge of the physiology of lactation and infant feeding to support effective management of challenges that might arise at any time during breastfeeding
- Have an understanding of the special circumstances which can affect lactation and breastfeeding and be able to support mothers to overcome the challenges
- Have the knowledge and skills to access the evidence that underpins infant feeding practice and know how to keep up to date

Tongue-tie – Ankyloglossia

Tongue-tie (Ankyloglossia) is a congenital anomaly in which the frenulum is shorter or thicker than usual and causes the infant's tongue to be retracted when normally it would extend over the lower lip when the mouth is opened wide (Genna 2013). Tongue-tie is more common in boys than girls, and the reported incidence varies from 3% to 10% (Baker & Carr 2015; Henry & Hayman 2014). Whilst some infants with tongue-tie can breastfeed normally, others are unable to attach to the breast properly and this may lead to sore nipples (Jamilian et al 2014). As the anterior tongue is used to stabilize the breast and suction coupled with wave-like movements of the tongue transfers milk into the baby's mouth, inefficient milk transfer may result, leading to an unsettled baby and poor weight gain. Bottle feeding may also be difficult for some infants with tongue-tie.

If a baby is having difficulty attaching to the breast, then the baby should be closely observed whilst feeding. Often a baby with tongue-tie will try to latch but will repeatedly pull away from the breast (Henry & Hayman 2014). Some of the signs that might be apparent are presented in Table 8.1.

If the tongue-tie means the baby is not able to feed, division can be performed by a trained healthcare professional, usually in early infancy. The baby's head is stabilized and the frenulum is divided using sharp blunt-ended scissors. This is not usually painful, does not bleed much and the baby is able to feed immediately after the procedure (National Institute for Health and Clinical Excellence 2005). Limited evidence suggests this improves the baby's ability to breastfeed in most cases (Ito 2014; National Institute for Health and Clinical Excellence 2005).

Table 8.1 **Signs of a tongue-tie**

Maternal issues	Infant issues
Sore or damaged nipples	Difficulty latching onto breast
Nipples flattened after feed	Unable to create/maintain suction
Concern about milk supply	Slipping off breast during a feed
Mastitis	Clicking sound whilst feeding
Mother may become frustrated	Poor milk transfer
May want to give up breastfeeding	Poor weight gain
	Frequent and/or prolonged feeds

Sources (Genna 2013; Henry & Hayman 2014).

Cleft lip and palate

Cleft palate is a structural gap in the roof of the baby's mouth, either in the hard or the soft palate or both and may be accompanied by a cleft lip. The incidence is around 1.7 per 1000 births in the UK (Mossey et al 2009). Babies with clefts may have problems feeding because they have difficulties creating a good seal to produce suction, which is essential for breastfeeding and bottle feeding. If a baby has only a cleft lip or a small or narrow cleft palate, they may be able to breastfeed although the mother may need to try different positions. A study in Scotland found that 80% of babies with cleft lip breastfed initially and 67% of these were still breastfeeding at 6 months (Britton et al 2011). However, babies with cleft palate or bilateral cleft lip were less likely to be breastfed (Britton et al 2011). Often, an upright position for breastfeeding may be most successful; the mother may need to position the baby to occlude the cleft with the breast tissue and may need extra support.

Breast milk is optimal for babies with clefts as these babies often have milk in their nasal cavity and breast milk is less irritating to the mucous membranes than formula; it also helps prevent ear and nasal infections. These babies also have a tendency to swallow air and often experience fatigue trying to suckle. Careful monitoring of weight gain is needed and supplementation of expressed breast milk may be necessary (Martin & Greatrex-White 2014). Clefts are sometimes, but not always, diagnosed antenatally at the 20-week scan. If identified, this can help to prepare parents psychologically before birth, and counselling will be advantageous (Goodacre & Swan 2008). After birth, the family will require specialist help and support from a multi-professional team.

Hypoglycaemia

Babies, like all mammalian newborns, have low blood glucose concentrations 1 to 2 hours after birth as they make the transition to extra-uterine life. Most newborns compensate through a process known as counterregulation, by producing alternative fuels. For example, they release glycogen from body stores to produce glucose and mobilize ketones from fat (Adamkin & Committee on Fetus and Newborn 2011; Walker 2017). This natural fall in blood glucose concentration means it is not helpful to routinely measure blood glucose in asymptomatic babies who are under 2 hours of age even if they have not fed as this will lead to unnecessary intervention. Breastfed babies generally have lower plasma glucose concentrations but a higher concentration of ketones than formula-fed babies (Adamkin & Committee on Fetus and Newborn 2011). Breast milk is more ketogenic than formula (i.e. it promotes the production of ketones as an alternative brain fuel; Walker 2017) and it is this increased production of ketones that may enable breastfed babies to cope with lower levels of glucose.

It is important to recognize babies who may be 'at risk' of hypoglycaemia because symptomatic hypoglycaemia can lead to neurological injury if not treated appropriately. Risk factors include: small or large for gestational age, prematurity, asphyxia and/or respiratory distress, infection, inborn errors of metabolism, diabetic mother, cold stress after birth, use of intravenous dextrose in labour and maternal drugs that affect glucose status (e.g. tocolytics, beta blockers such as Labetalol; Pollard 2012; Walker 2017). It is also crucial to recognize the signs and symptoms of neonatal hypoglycaemia such as: lethargy, irritability, altered level of consciousness, apnoea, cyanosis, hypothermia or convulsions (Pollard 2012; UNICEF Baby Friendly Initiative UK 2011).

Prevention is the goal and some of the practice recommendations for babies at risk of hypoglycaemia are similar to recommendations for all babies such as encouraging skin-to-skin contact to maintain the baby's body temperature, regulate heart rate, reduce stress, crying and encourage early and frequent breastfeeding. Early breastfeeding will help to mobilize alternative energy sources and stabilization of vital signs, and reduction of stress will lead to reduced energy expenditure. In addition, infants with higher risk of hypoglycaemia will require regular monitoring of vital signs and blood glucose. There is no agreed level of plasma glucose concentration or duration of hypoglycaemia that is associated with clinical signs or permanent neurological injury, so there are variations in local guidelines (Adamkin & Committee on Fetus and Newborn 2011; UNICEF Baby Friendly Initiative UK 2011). If an infant is symptomatic or screening reveals low blood glucose, breastfed infants should be offered expressed colostrum via a cup, syringe or nasogastric tube and formula-fed infants should also have frequent effective feeds. Some infants may require intravenous fluids.

Activity

Access the guideline for care of a baby with hypoglycaemia in your area of work. At what level in the first 24 hours would a baby be considered to be hypoglycaemic? Download the UNICEF BFI guidance for developing a policy for the prevention and management of hypoglycaemia of the newborn at http://www.unicef.org.uk/BabyFriendly/Resources/Guidance-for-Health-Professionals/Writing-policies-and-guidelines/Hypoglycaemia-policy-guidelines/. Compare the sample flow chart for the management of breastfed babies at risk of hypoglycaemia with the guidance in your place of work.

Jaundice

Around 60% to 70% of babies become jaundiced (yellow pigment in the skin) in the first week of life (NICE 2010). This is caused by a breakdown of excess red blood cells as part of the neonate's response to extra-uterine life. The products of haemoglobin that break down are iron and un-conjugated bilirubin, which are processed by the liver. In a healthy term neonate, this normal physiological process does not usually pose any threat to health and, in most babies, a mild jaundice resolves spontaneously. For an explanation of the full process of breakdown of red blood cells, see Baston (2012). Usually Bilirubin levels increase gradually after birth and peak around 96 to 120 hours after birth and, for most infants, the condition resolves over the first week or two (Walker 2017). However, because high levels of bilirubin are toxic to the infant's brain and can cause a condition known as *Kernicterus*, careful monitoring is important. Kernicterus is the presence of bilirubin in the infant's brain tissues and can cause damage to the brain. It is not commonly seen in the UK; there are fewer than seven cases per year, and with improved care, it should become a condition of the past (The Lancet 2010).

Babies with physiological jaundice tend to be sleepy and often do not feed well, but the jaundice can become worse if the baby does not receive sufficient fluid and nutrition. Therefore mothers should be encouraged to cuddle the baby skin-to-skin and offer frequent access to the breast, being alert to the baby's feeding cues. The baby should be observed breastfeeding to ensure effective feeding and suggestions offered to ensure optimal positioning and attachment if necessary. If the baby does not feed regularly or effectively, breast milk expression may be required and offered by cup or spoon (Pollard 2012).

Other forms of jaundice include pathological jaundice and breast milk jaundice. Pathological jaundice occurs within the first 24 hours as a result of an underlying condition such as sepsis or rhesus incompatibility. It is always serious and requires medical review (NICE 2010). Breast milk jaundice generally occurs later, and the baby is usually alert and appears well. This type of jaundice can last some time, and it is not usually problematic. The association between breastfeeding and jaundice is not well understood and further research is needed to fully understand this (NICE 2010). However, assessment of bilirubin levels should be carried out and medical review is needed to exclude underlying medical conditions.

Activity

Consider and list the signs of ineffective milk transfer to a breastfed baby. What effect does a delay in passing meconium have on a baby? If a baby is becoming jaundiced, what percentage weight loss is acceptable?

REFLECTION ON THE TRIGGER SCENARIO

Look back at the trigger scenario.

> *Laura was born during the night and is now lying on her mother's chest. She has started to stir and is beginning to move her head from side-to-side. Her mother, Bethany, looks down at her and smiles. Laura has been very sleepy since birth and only made a few attempts to suckle despite lying against her mother skin-to-skin most of the time since her birth. 'Come on Laura,' she said, 'you must be hungry now.'*

Laura is sleepy and reluctant to feed in the early postnatal period. Bethany is holding her skin-to-skin and looking for feeding cues. Consider possible causes of Laura's reluctance to feed. What information and support might her mother need in the near future to continue to breastfeed?

This scenario highlights the challenge of identifying why a newborn baby might initially be reluctant to feed. Now that you are familiar with some of the baby-related issues that might affect breastfeeding, you should have insight into how the scenario relates to the evidence. The jigsaw model will now be used to explore the trigger scenario in more depth.

Effective communication

Women whose babies are reluctant to breastfeed initially after birth can become very concerned about this. It is therefore crucial that midwives and others supporting women experiencing this communicate sensitively with them. Midwives will need to consider underlying conditions, such as those discussed in this chapter; however at this early stage, women whose babies do not feed easily are most likely to need reassurance to build their confidence in their ability to breastfeed their baby. Questions that arise from the scenario might include: How might the midwife caring for Bethany reassure her? What verbal and non-verbal ways of communicating might the midwife use to do this? How might the midwife encourage Bethany to express her concerns? How can the midwife draw on the positive things Bethany has already done, such as provide skin-to-skin contact, to communicate in a way that starts to build her confidence?

Woman-centred care

For the midwife to care for Bethany and Laura effectively, she will need to be aware of their individual circumstances. Questions that arise from the scenario might include: Did anything happen during labour and/or birth that might have some effect on breastfeeding? Has a full neonatal examination been carried out after birth? If so, was anything highlighted from this that might provide an explanation for Laura's reluctance to feed? Has the midwife assessed Laura's condition recently? If so, is she a good colour and breathing normally? Might a structural anomaly, such as cleft palate, have been missed on a previous examination? Is Laura showing any signs of jaundice at this early stage? If so, what would the midwife do immediately?

Using best evidence

In this scenario, the evidence the midwife would need to draw on will depend on the likely cause of Laura's reluctance to feed. Healthy term babies often do not feed frequently in the first 24 to 48 hours and most can mobilize energy stores through counterregulation. These babies do not suffer ill effects from this unless the situation continues. With skilled support, most babies can and will breastfeed. However it is important that the midwife recognizes any factors that mean the baby may be at higher risk; in such cases, different management will be required. Questions that arise from the scenario might include: Is Laura at risk of hypoglycaemia for any reason? Laura is likely to be warm as she is lying in skin-to-skin contact with Bethany; is she also covered with a baby blanket? If Laura was to get cold, what effect might this have? If Laura continues to be sleepy and reluctant to breastfeed, what might you do that would mean that Laura gets some breast milk and may also encourage Bethany to continue to breastfeed?

Professional and legal issues

Midwives should work collaboratively with other members of the healthcare team respecting the skills and expertise of their colleagues (NMC 2015). Laura may simply be reluctant to feed, and this may be resolved with sensitive support. If, however, a congenital condition is identified or she develops a condition such as hypoglycaemia or jaundice, the midwife should involve other professionals and a team approach to care would be essential. Questions that arise from the scenario might include: Who might the midwife involve in the care of Laura and Bethany if a congenital condition is identified? Who might the midwife approach if Laura continues to be reluctant to feed? Which national or local guidelines might the midwife need to access? How would the care provided for Laura and Bethany be documented?

Team working

Most women who have a baby who is reluctant to feed initially after birth will be supported by a midwife. As time progresses, if the baby still does not feed, the midwife may need to liaise with others. Some Trusts have lactation consultants who can be contacted for further expert support and, in some areas, lactation consultants are qualified to carry out division of tongue-tie. The midwife caring for Bethany and Laura may also involve the paediatrician if, for example, there is concern about an underlying health condition, the baby is at high risk of either hypo-glycaemia or appears jaundiced within 24 hours after birth. Although relatively uncommon, if a baby is found to have a congenital structural anomaly such as a cleft requiring surgical treatment, effective high-quality care will require consultation and support from a multi-professional team. Questions that arise from the scenario might include: If the midwife caring for Bethany decided to contact the lactation consultant, what aspects of Bethany and Laura's clinical histories might need to be explained? How would this have been recorded in the clinical records? What might the lactation consultant do first? How would the midwife decide if and when to involve a paediatrician?

Clinical dexterity

To provide sensitive support for Bethany, effective communication skills are essential; however, in this scenario, good clinical skills are also needed. These might include aspects such as observational skills to identify when the baby is likely to feed so that opportunities to provide timely support are not missed. Once Laura attempts to feed, recognition of good attachment will be necessary. Knowledge of positions that might encourage her to feed most effectively would also be helpful. If Laura continues to be reluctant to feed, observational skills would be needed to identify why this might be. Knowledge of babies who are likely to be at risk would also help the midwife to make a timely referral to a paediatrician if required. Questions that arise from the scenario might include: Is Laura displaying any cues that she is ready to feed? How would the lactation consultant be contacted in your area of work? Is Laura showing any signs of respiratory distress? Has the midwife examined Laura thoroughly?

Models of care

Models of care that provide continuity of care are likely to be most helpful to mothers like Bethany as conflicting advice is often a concern for breastfeeding women, particularly in the early days and in the hospital setting (Dykes 2006; Marshall et al 2007). This can undermine women's confidence in their ability to feed their baby and may lead them to decide to stop breastfeeding. In this scenario, questions that might arise include: Where are Bethany and Laura receiving care? Are they likely to receive consistent advice and support? Midwife-led models of care might be more likely to provide continuity of care, but what would need to happen if a referral to a paediatrician was required? If support from a lactation consultant was provided, is it likely that Bethany would have met her before?

Safe environment

To provide safe care for Bethany and Laura, it will be essential to spend time observing Laura's behaviour and clinical condition to rule out or identify any potential problems as early as possible. For example, recognizing if Laura is at higher risk of hypoglycaemia or jaundice can lead to prompt management and will therefore enhance safety by preventing sequelae such as neurological damage. Questions that arise from the scenario might include: What is the guidance for care of babies with hypoglycaemia in your area of work? What is the guidance for care of babies with jaundice under 24 hours old? Access the NICE guideline. Are there any differences between the guideline in your area and NICE guidance?

Promotes health

Breastfeeding can protect babies against many diseases and conditions, and the evidence for this is gradually increasing (Hoddinott et al 2008;

Rollins et al 2016; Victora et al 2016). Therefore making sufficient time to provide adequate, sensitive support for mothers and babies in the early days after birth has the potential to promote health across generations. If conditions such as those discussed in this chapter are identified, breast milk can be even more beneficial to the baby's health; for example, if a baby with a cleft is able to breastfeed, they will be better protected against infection and therefore less likely to have ear or respiratory infections. If a baby remains unable to breastfeed, a mother may wish to give her baby expressed breast milk. Colostrum is calorie rich, so a few millilitres will start to raise Laura's blood glucose levels. Extra support and different feeding positions may be needed to achieve these outcomes. Questions that might arise from the scenario include: If Bethany was to express some colostrum, how would she do so at this early stage? How could this be given to Laura to optimize breastfeeding in the future? What living components are there in colostrum that quickly confers health benefits to babies such as Laura? Approximately what quantity of colostrum is Laura likely to need at each feed in the first 24 hours? How might you visually demonstrate this to Bethany?

Further scenarios

The following scenarios enable you to consider how specific situations influence the care the midwife provides. Use the jigsaw model to explore the issues raised in each situation.

SCENARIO 1

Heidi had her baby, Joshua, 5 days ago. Joshua is Heidi's second baby, and he was born in the local birth centre. Joshua breastfed well initially after birth and has fed eagerly and often at home during the first few days. When he was 3 days old, he started to become jaundiced, sleepy and less eager to feed. Pat, the community midwife, has just arrived to see them both and asks Heidi how things are going now.

Practice point

Physiological jaundice is the most common type. It is usually self-limiting and does not normally cause any lasting problems for the baby. The NICE postnatal guideline states that the mother of a jaundiced breastfed baby should be encouraged to feed often and should not routinely be given extra fluids or formula. 'If the baby appears significantly jaundiced or seems unwell then evaluation of serum bilirubin level should be carried out' (NICE 2006:30).

Further points specific to Scenario 1 include:

1. What questions might the midwife, Pat, ask Heidi?
2. Why might a mother with a jaundiced baby need more support to breastfeed?
3. What might Pat suggest to Heidi to encourage and enable her to breastfeed more often?
4. How are serum bilirubin levels in babies evaluated and measured in your area of work?
5. What are the risks to Joshua if his serum bilirubin levels were to become high?
6. Look at the NICE guideline for jaundice in newborn babies under 28 days old (NICE 2010). What factors would indicate a higher risk of Kernicterus?

SCENARIO 2

Maryam's baby, Akbar, was born with a unilateral cleft lip. Immediately after birth, Maryam was upset but they are now on the postnatal ward and the midwife is providing support to Maryam to breastfeed Akbar.

Practice point

Clefts are not always identified on scan during pregnancy so mothers may not be prepared when their baby is born. A cleft lip occurs during the fifth to eighth week of pregnancy when the two sides of the lip do not fuse properly. A cleft lip, because it is clearly visible, may be particularly psychologically distressing for parents, so sensitive support is likely to be needed. As discussed earlier, most babies with a cleft lip will be able to breastfeed (Britton et al 2011) but some adjustments, such as extra support and different feeding positions, may be needed. A baby with cleft lip and/or palate is likely to tire easily whilst feeding so they may need supplementary feeding with expressed breast milk (Walker 2017).

Further points specific to Scenario 2 include:

1. What would you say to Maryam had you been present at the birth?
2. What feeding positions might be most effective for a baby with a cleft lip?
3. When a baby is feeding, suction is needed in the oral cavity for the baby to stay on the breast and for milk removal (Ramsey et al 2005). What might the mother be advised to do to help the baby achieve this?
4. What other members of the multi-disciplinary team might be involved in the early care of Akbar and Maryam?
5. What kind of specialist support might be needed?

Conclusion

When a baby is reluctant to feed, this is a source of concern for the mother and healthcare professionals. Understanding the physiology of the baby's adaptation to extra-uterine life, including how babies mobilize other energy sources at this time, can prevent unnecessary intervention. Whilst most babies only require time with their mother in skin-to-skin contact and sensitive support to initiate breastfeeding, midwives have an important role to play in terms of recognizing when a baby is ill, has a congenital disorder or a physiological condition such as jaundice and managing this in a way that is supportive of a mother's wish to breastfeed.

Resources

BAPRAS website. Available at: http://www.bapras.org.uk/public/patient-information/surgery-guides/cleft-lip-and-palate.

BFI guidance for developing a policy for the prevention and management of hypoglycaemia of the newborn. Available at: http://www.unicef.org.uk/BabyFriendly/Resources/Guidance-for-Health-Professionals/Writing-policies-and-guidelines/Hypoglycaemia-policy-guidelines/.

CLAPA website. Available at: https://www.clapa.com/.

National Institute for Health and Clinical Excellence, 2005. *Division of Ankyloglossia (Tongue-Tie) for Breastfeeding*. National Institute for Health and Clinical Excellence, London. Available at: https://www.nice.org.uk/guidance/IPG149/chapter/2-The-procedure.

NICE, 2010. Jaundice in Newborn Babies Under 28 Days. *Clinical Guideline 98*. National Collaborating Centre for Women's and Children's Health, London. Available at: https://www.nice.org.uk/guidance/cg98/resources/jaundice-in-newborn-babies-under-28-days-975756073669.

References

Adamkin, D.H., Committee on Fetus and Newborn, 2011. Postnatal glucose homeostasis in late-preterm and term infants. Pediatrics 127, 575–579.

Baker, A.R., Carr, M.M., 2015. Surgical treatment of ankyloglossia. Oper. Tech. Otolaryngol. Head Neck Surg. 26, 28–32.

Baston, H., 2012. Use of technology in childbirth: 6. Phototherapy. Pract. Midwife 15, 36–39.

Britton, K.F.M., McDonald, S.H., Welbury, R.R., 2011. An investigation into infant feeding in children born with a cleft lip and/or palate in the West of Scotland. Eur. Arch. Paediatr. Dent. 12, 250–255.

Colson, S.D., Meek, J.H., Hawdon, J.M., 2008. Optimal positions for the release of primitive neonatal reflexes stimulating breastfeeding. Early Hum. Dev. 84, 441–449.

Dykes, F., 2006. Breastfeeding in Hospital: Mothers, Midwives and The Production Line. Routledge, Abingdon.

Genna, C.W., 2013. The influence of anatomic and structural issues on sucking skills. In: Genna, C.W. (Ed.), Supporting Suckling Skills in Breastfeeding Infants, second ed. Jones and Bartlett, New York.

Genna, C.W., Sandora, L., 2013. Breastfeeding: normal sucking and swallowing. In: Supporting Suckling Skills in Breastfeeding Infants. Jones and Bartlett, New York.

Goodacre, T., Swan, M.C., 2008. Cleft lip and palate: current management. Paediatr. Child Health 18, 283–292.

Henry, L., Hayman, R., 2014. Ankyloglossia - Its Impact Breastfeeding. Nurs. Womens Health 18, 122–129.

Hoddinott, P., Tappin, D., Wright, C., 2008. Breast feeding. BMJ 336, 881–887.

Ito, Y., 2014. Does frenotomy improve breast-feeding difficulties in infants with ankyloglossia? Frenotomy in infants with ankyloglossia. Pediatr. Int. 56, 497–505.

Jamilian, A., Fattahi, F.H., Kootanayi, N.G., 2014. Ankyloglossia and tongue mobility. Eur. Arch. Paediatr. Dent. 15, 33–35.

Marshall, J.L., Godfrey, M., Renfrew, M.J., 2007. Being a 'good mother': Managing breastfeeding and merging identities. Soc. Sci. Med. 65, 2147–2159.

Martin, V., Greatrex-White, S., 2014. An evaluation of factors influencing feeding in babies with a cleft palate with and without a cleft lip. J. Child Health Care 18, 72–83.

McAndrew, F., Thompson, J., Fellows, L., et al., 2012. Infant Feeding Survey 2010. Health and Social Care Information Centre, London.

Mossey, P.A., Little, J., Munger, R.G., et al., 2009. Cleft lip and palate. Lancet 374, 1773–1785.

National Institute for Health and Clinical Excellence, 2005. Division of Ankyloglossia (Tongue-Tie) for Breastfeeding. National Institute for Health and Clinical Excellence, London.

NICE, 2006. Routine Postnatal Care of Women and Their Babies. NICE, London.

NICE, 2010. *Jaundice in Newborn Babies Under 28 Days*. Clinical Guideline 98. National Collaborating Centre for Women's and Children's Health, London.

NMC, 2015. The Code: Professional Standards of Practice and Behaviour for Nurses and Midwives. Nursing and Midwifery Council., London. Available at: https://www.nmc.org.uk/globalassets/sitedocuments/nmc-publications/nmc-code.pdf.

Pollard, M., 2012. Evidence-Based Care for Breastfeeding Mothers. Routledge, London.

Ramsey, D.T., Kent, R.A., Hartmann, R.A., Hartmann, P.E., 2005. Anatomy of the lactating human breast redefined with ultrasound imaging. J. Anat. 206, 525–534.

Rollins, N.C., Bhandari, N., Hajeebhoy, N., et al., 2016. Why invest, and what it will take to improve breastfeeding practices? Lancet 387, 491–504.

The Lancet, 2010. Detection and treatment of neonatal jaundice. Lancet 375, 1845.

UNICEF Baby Friendly Initiative UK, 2011. Guidance on the Development of Policies and Guidelines for the Prevention and Management of Hypoglycaemia of the Newborn. UNICEF Baby Friendly Initiative, London. Available at: http://www.unicef.org.uk/Documents/Baby_Friendly/Guidance/4/hypo_policy.pdf?epslanguage=en. (Accessed 16 December 2012).

Victora, C.G., Bahl, R., Barros, A.J.D., et al., 2016. Breastfeeding in the 21st century: epidemiology, mechanisms, and lifelong effect. Lancet 387, 475–490.

Walker, M., 2017. Breastfeeding Management for the Clinician: Using the Evidence, fourth ed. Jones and Bartlett, Burlington.

CHAPTER 9

Formula feeding

TRIGGER SCENARIO

Sadie is breastfeeding her baby, Tom. She has recently had a visit from her mother who has undermined her confidence by telling her that she is 'probably not feeding Tom enough or that her milk is not strong enough' because he is feeding often. Sadie is now not sure whether to carry on breastfeeding – after all, she and her three brothers are all very healthy and they were all fed formula. She looks down at baby Tom who is lying in her arms gazing up at her face and says 'I just want you to grow, be strong, healthy and happy'. Sadie decides she will ask the community midwife when she visits later in the day.

Introduction

Most parents have one thing in common – they all want their children to be healthy and happy, and in the early days after birth, infant feeding is a major part of the care of the baby as women make the transition to motherhood. However women choose to feed their baby, they like to think they are doing the right thing for both their baby and themselves. Although women have breastfed their babies for millions of years, and it is after all what defines us as mammals, in the 21st century in many countries, bottle feeding with formula has become so common that it is perceived by many people as the normal way to feed babies. Every day worldwide, women make choices about infant feeding, and these choices should be underpinned by accurate knowledge so that women and families can evaluate risks and benefits of the different options. Whilst formula may be nutritionally adequate for growth of human babies, it cannot be considered to be equivalent to breast milk. Breast milk is much more than nutrition; it is a dynamic, complex living fluid that both nourishes and protects against disease as it has all the nutrients for optimal growth and development, a host of immunological factors such as macrophages and lymphocytes and transfer factors that aid the digestion of micronutrients such as iron.

UNICEF Baby Friendly Maternity Standards

The following are the maternity standards that are most relevant to this chapter:

- Support all mothers and babies to initiate a close relationship and feeding soon after birth
- Support mothers to make informed decisions regarding the introduction of food or fluids other than breast milk

UNICEF Baby Friendly UK University Learning Outcomes

The following are the learning outcomes that are achieved within this chapter. By the end of their midwifery education programme, students will:

- Appreciate the importance of breast milk and breastfeeding on the health and wellbeing of mothers and babies
- Draw on their knowledge and understanding of the wider social, cultural and political influences which undermine breastfeeding, to promote, support and protect breastfeeding within their sphere of practice
- Have the knowledge and skills to access the evidence that underpins infant feeding practice and know how to keep up to date

The neonate's gut and infant feeding

Colonization of the neonate's gut with bacteria is a complex process. It used to be thought that, before birth, a baby's gut is sterile, but more recent research has demonstrated the presence of bacteria in the meconium of term infants (Jiménez et al 2008). This suggests that infants may develop their first gut microbiome in utero. Bacteria from the mother's gut appears to reach the amniotic fluid via the blood stream, and colonization occurs as the fetus swallows (Jiménez et al 2008). This bacterial colonization then continues during birth and afterward throughout feeding. The infant's gut microbiome is affected by a range of factors but primarily the mode of birth and type of infant feeding (Penders et al 2006). If a baby is born vaginally, the gut is colonized by bacteria from the mother; however, if a baby is born by caesarean their gut is more likely to become colonized with bacteria from the environment (Walker 2013). In addition to this, more recent research suggests that the gut flora may be modified by factors such as physiological stress or hormonal signals during labour, maternal obesity and antibiotic use (Azad et al 2016; Cabrera-Rubio et al 2012).

After birth, infant feeding has a major role to play. Breast milk contains a rich diversity of beneficial bacteria, and colostrum has a higher diversity than mature milk (Cabrera-Rubio et al 2012). Intestinal bacteria are important to health as they provide a barrier to the colonization of pathogens and they stimulate the development of an infant's immune system (Penders et al 2006). The gut microbiome also influences metabolism and therefore, along with epigenetic modifications, plays a part in future health (Aaltonen et al 2011; Neu 2016).

There are major differences in the gut flora of breastfed and formula-fed infants. When a baby is breastfed, the gut is much more acidic (pH of 5.1–5.4 compared with 5.9–7.3 in formula-fed infants), has high levels of *Bifidobacterium* which are important beneficial bacteria and fewer potentially harmful bacteria such as *E. coli*, and *Streptococci* (Morelli 2008; Walker 2013). When infants are given supplements of formula during the first 7 days of life, the infant's gut becomes more like the gut of a formula-fed infant in that the gut becomes more alkaline and the percentage of *Bifidobacterium* decreases (Walker 2013). At birth, an infant's gut mucosa is immature and the intestine is permeable to proteins and pathogens. The process of maturation takes many weeks but occurs much more quickly when an infant is exclusively breastfed. Antibodies in colostrum and breast milk coat the gut providing protection whilst the gut is immature (Walker 2013). Mothers produce specific antibodies when they either ingest or inhale pathogens, and when an infant breastfeeds, these are ingested and will bind to the pathogen in the infant's gut to prevent disease. Therefore if mother and baby stay together, they will be exposed to the same pathogens and the baby will be protected. However, feeding formula to a baby interferes with this mechanism, and the baby is then not protected in this way (Walker 2013).

The risks of formula feeding

Babies in developing countries who are not breastfed are likely to be less healthy and have a higher risk of dying in infancy (Victora et al 2016; WHO Collaborative Study Team on the Role of Breastfeeding on the Prevention of Infant Mortality 2000). This has recently been found to be the case in high income countries in relation to unexplained infant death (Victora et al 2016). Most women in the UK (82%) are aware of at least some of the short- and long-term health consequences for babies who are not breastfed (McAndrew et al 2012). These include a higher risk of being ill with diarrhoea, otitis media or lower respiratory tract infections (Ip et al 2009; Quigley et al 2007). Quigley et al (2007) measured the effects of breastfeeding on admissions to hospital using the Millennium Cohort Study (15,890 healthy singleton term infants born in 2000–2002) and estimated that 53% of hospitalizations for diarrhoea and 27% for lower respiratory tract infections could have been prevented each month if all infants were exclusively breastfed.

Several reviews of the evidence for longer-term health outcomes for both mother and baby have been conducted. These suggest that not breastfeeding increases a mother's risk of developing breast cancer, ovarian cancer, type 2 diabetes and postnatal depression (Hoddinott et al 2008; Victora et al 2016). Infants who are not breastfed may have increased risk of high blood pressure, obesity, type 1 and type 2 diabetes, childhood leukaemia, sudden infant death syndrome, necrotizing enterocolitis and atopic dermatitis and asthma (Hoddinott et al 2008; Ip et al 2009). However, a recent international review did not find clear evidence of an association between breastfeeding and allergic disease, such as asthma and eczema (Victora et al 2016). But, after adjusting for confounding factors such as socioeconomic status, this study did find a consistent association between breastfeeding and higher results in intelligence tests and lower rates of childhood leukaemia (Victora et al 2016).

Activity

Consider what information about breastfeeding and formula feeding women might be most interested to know. Do you think this is most likely to be health related? Access a website such as www.mumsnet.com and have a look at the conversations about infant feeding choices and support. Consider how you can provide accurate information about infant feeding in a way that is helpful to women.

Trends in infant feeding in the UK

The World Health Organization (WHO) recommends that women continue to breastfeed their infants for 2 years having exclusively breastfed for 6 months (World Health Organization 2003). Breastfeeding rates in the UK are amongst the lowest in Europe, and the most recent infant feeding survey showed that, although more women were breastfeeding at all time points in the UK, only just over a third (34%) were breastfeeding when their baby was 6 months of age (McAndrew et al 2012). Only 23% of women were exclusively breastfeeding when the baby was 6 weeks old (McAndrew et al 2012).

More women in managerial and professional occupations, those over 30 and those who left education after 18 years choose to breastfeed their babies (McAndrew et al 2012) – a continuing trend noted in previous infant feeding surveys (e.g. Bolling et al 2007). This has changed over time however, as prior to the industrial revolution more women from lower social classes breastfed (Palmer 2009).

Formula feeding

Some women choose to feed their baby formula milk for a variety of reasons, and just a few women are not able to breastfeed; it is important that these women are given the information they need and feel well supported. This involves showing mothers how to sterilize feeding equipment effectively and how to make up a formula feed correctly.

Most formula milks are made from cows' milk and are modified to make them suitable for babies. A range of different milks is available, and it is important that parents know which one is suitable for their baby at which age. First milks are for newborn babies and are whey-based to aid digestion (whey:casein ratio is 60:40; Crawley & Westland 2016). When a mother has chosen not to breastfeed, first milk should be fed to a baby until 5 months of age and can be continued as solids are introduced until the infant is 1 year. Formula milks marketed for hungrier babies are casein dominant (whey:casein ratio is 20:80) and are therefore more difficult to digest. Although these are marketed for hungry babies, there is no evidence of benefit over standard first milks (Crawley & Westland 2016). Follow-on milks are marketed for babies over 6 months (and must not be given to babies before 6 months), but there is no evidence of any benefits to infants from having this milk rather than first milk so these milks are not recommended (Crawley & Westland 2016; UNICEF Baby Friendly UK & First Steps Nutrition Trust 2016).

The 2010 Infant Feeding Survey demonstrated that less than half of mothers in the UK made formula feeds as recommended – that is, only making one feed at a time, making feeds within 30 minutes of the water boiling and putting the water into the bottle before the powder (McAndrew et al 2012). This suggests that women may not always be given the information they need to ensure safe formula feeding.

Making up a formula feed

Parents who are formula feeding will need to know what equipment to buy and how to sterilize this for feeding. They will also need to understand how to make up feeds in line with current guidance and how to feed their baby safely. The following instructions are from the leaflet produced jointly by UNICEF Baby Friendly and the Department of Health (UNICEF Baby Friendly Initiative UK & Department of Health 2013).

Equipment needed

To feed a baby formula milk, parents will need bottles with teats and bottle covers, bottle brush and teat brush, formula milk powder or ready-to-feed formula and a sterilizing unit (either a steam sterilizer, a cold-water sterilizing solution or sterilizing by boiling).

How to sterilize equipment

Equipment to be used for either formula milk or expressed breast milk should be sterilized. First, the person preparing the feed should wash their hands. Then all items of equipment should be cleaned before sterilizing by washing thoroughly in hot soapy water and then rinsed in cold running water. There are three main methods of sterilizing equipment.

If using a cold-water sterilizing solution:

+ The manufacturer's instructions should be followed
+ The solution should be changed every 24 hours
+ Equipment should be left in the solution for at least 30 minutes
+ There should be no air trapped in any of the bottles or teats

If using a steam sterilizer:

+ There are different types of steam sterilizers so it is very important to follow the manufacturer's instructions
+ The openings of the bottles and teats should be facing down in the sterilizer
+ Manufacturers will provide instructions as to how long the equipment can be left after sterilizing, if it is not used straight away, before it needs to be resterillized

If sterilizing using boiling:

+ Safety should be maintained. Boiling pans should not be left unattended especially if there are children in the vicinity
+ Any equipment to be sterilized this way should be safe to be boiled (teats tend to become damaged more easily when boiled)
+ Equipment should be boiled for 10 minutes ensuring that it stays under the water

When putting teats and bottles together, hands should be washed and the surface to be used should be clean and disinfected. The bottles should be removed just before they are used and, if they are not to be used immediately, should be put together with the teat and lid in place to prevent the inside of the bottle or the teat from becoming contaminated.

Activity

Access the Internet and explore the range of sterilizers. Prepare a list and make some notes on each. There are some machines available that make up formula feeds. Using the Internet, check out the range of these and how they work.

How to make up a feed

Parents need to understand that good hygiene is important when making up bottle feeds and that this is because babies are more susceptible to illness and infection as their immune system is not as well developed as an adult's immune system. It is therefore crucial that parents understand the need to sterilize all equipment as previously explained. They also need to know that formula powder is not sterile even when the tins are sealed and that, although rare, formula can contain harmful bacteria that can cause serious illness. To avoid this happening, it should be explained to parents that they should make up each feed as the baby needs it using boiled water at 70°C or above. Fresh drinking water from the tap should be boiled rather than bottled, softened or previously boiled water as the balance of minerals in these types of water may not be suitable for making up formula feed as there may be too much sodium or sulphate.

A step-by-step process for making up a bottle feed should be explained to parents as follows. Parents need to know they should:

1. Fill the kettle with at least 1 litre of **fresh tap water from the cold tap** (they need to know they should not use water that has been boiled before).
2. Boil the water. Then leave the water to cool in the kettle for **no more than 30 minutes so that it remains at a temperature of at least 70°C.**
3. Clean and disinfect the surface they are going to use.
4. It's really important to emphasize that they should **WASH THEIR HANDS**.
5. If they are using a cold-water sterilizer, shake off any excess solution from the bottle and the teat, or rinse the bottle with cooled boiled water from the kettle (not the tap).
6. Stand the bottle on a clean surface.
7. Keep the teat and cap on the upturned lid of the sterilizer. Avoid putting them on the work surface.
8. Follow the manufacturer's instructions and pour the correct amount of water into the bottle. Double check that the water level is correct. It is really important that parents have understood the need to put the water in the bottle first, while it is still hot, before adding the powdered infant formula.
9. Loosely fill the scoop with formula – according to the manufacturer's instructions – and level it off using either the flat edge of a clean, dry knife or the leveller provided. It is crucial that parents realize the importance of using the correct amount of powder and that different types of formula come with different-sized scoops. Using

too much formula could make their baby ill, cause constipation or dehydration and using too little would lead to poor nourishment and less than optimal weight gain.

10. Holding the edge of the teat, put it on the bottle. Then screw the retaining ring onto the bottle.

11. Cover the teat with the cap and shake the bottle until the powder is dissolved.

12. It is important to cool the formula so it is not too hot to drink. This can be done by holding the bottom half of the bottle under cold running water. Move the bottle about under the tap to ensure even cooling. Make sure that the water does not touch the cap covering the teat.

13. Test the temperature of the infant formula on the inside of their wrist before giving it to their baby. It should be body temperature, which means it should feel warm or cool, but not hot.

14. If there is any made-up infant formula left after a feed, parents need to know they should throw it away.

Ready-to-feed infant formula can be used, and this is sterile until opened. This is recommended for babies who may be vulnerable to infection, for example, if they are premature or small for gestational age. Ready-to-feed formula is generally more expensive than powdered formula but may be useful in certain circumstances such as when travelling. Parents will need to know that all equipment still needs to be sterilized and that they should follow the manufacturer's instructions. They also need to know that, once opened, ready-to-feed formula can be stored on the top shelf in the back of the fridge with the open corner turned down for a maximum of 24 hours.

It should be explained to parents that bacteria multiply quickly at room temperature so infant formula (either made from powder or the ready to feed type) that has not been used and has been kept at room temperature must be thrown away within 2 hours. Also that bacteria survive even at low temperatures in a fridge, although they will multiply more slowly in this environment.

Advising parents how to bottle feed responsively

It is crucial to have a conversation with parents about building a relationship with their baby. When women have chosen to formula feed it may be even more important to try to enhance the relationship they build with their baby (as discussed in Chapter 2). A key point is that the number of people who feed the baby should be limited to enable this to happen. It may be necessary to encourage women to think about feeding as a special time with their baby, to encourage them to make and maintain good eye contact and to stroke and caress their baby as this will help the baby to relax and feel safe. Skin-to-skin contact may also be helpful in this respect. Development of a loving and close relationship between parents and their baby help to ensure optimal brain development and can have long-ranging positive effects on the baby into childhood and adulthood (as explained in more detail in Chapter 2).

It is often assumed that parents will know how to bottle feed their baby, but this is not necessarily the case. When explaining this, in line with the UNICEF Baby Friendly and the Department of Health (UNICEF Baby Friendly Initiative UK & Department of Health 2013), a midwife can take the opportunity to encourage parents to hold their baby close, to touch them and to look into their eyes whilst they are feeding. It should be explained to parents that they should:

+ hold their baby fairly upright, with their head supported so that they can breathe and swallow comfortably
+ that they can brush the teat against the baby's mouth and when their baby opens their mouth, to allow them to draw in the teat
+ that if the teat becomes flattened while they are feeding, they can pull gently on the corner of their baby's mouth to release the vacuum
+ that their baby may need short breaks during the feed and may need to bring up wind
+ that when their baby does not want any more feed, to hold them upright and gently rub or pat their back to bring up any more wind
+ and crucially that they should take notice of their baby's cues that they have had enough milk and to avoid forcing their baby to take more than they want (UNICEF Baby Friendly Initiative UK & Department of Health 2013).

Parents will also need to know approximately how much to feed their baby and to understand that, although at first their baby may only take very small amounts this will increase throughout the first week. From the end of the first week, most babies will take around 150 to 200 ml per kg body weight per day. It is important to explain that babies do not necessarily feed in a regular pattern or take a regular amount and that they will need feeding at night. A discussion about recognizing their baby's feeding cues will be helpful. Encouraging parents to start feeding before their baby is crying is likely to mean that bottle feeding is easier.

Activity

Access the NCT explanation of what is in a baby's nappy at https://www.nct.org.uk/parenting/whats-your-babys-nappy. Might this help you to explain to a parent how they might know if their baby is feeding well? What other factors might help parents to know their baby is feeding enough?

The International Code of Marketing of Breastmilk Substitutes (the code)

The International Code of Marketing of Breastmilk Substitutes was adopted by the World Health Assembly in 1981 to protect and promote breastfeeding by providing adequate information on infant feeding and by the regulation of marketing of breast milk substitutes (World Health Organization 1981). It applies to governments and companies. The code advocates breastfeeding and, if babies are not breastfed, that they should be fed by the next best alternative. So formula should be available if needed but not be promoted. In summary: formula companies should not promote their products to the public, they should not provide free samples or gifts to mothers or to health workers, any information provided to health workers should be scientific and factual and not be misleading and all formula milk labels should state the benefits of breastfeeding and the risks of formula feeding and should not have pictures of babies or language that idealizes the use of the product.

Activity

Guidance has been produced for health workers to help them to use the code in their everyday practice with confidence. This can be accessed at https://www.unicef.org.uk/babyfriendly/baby-friendly-resources/guidance-for-health-professionals/the-code/a-guide-for-health-workers-to-working-within-the-international-code-of-marketing-of-breastmilk-substitutes/. Consider how advertising influences the behaviour of health professionals and what impact this might have on parents. Ensure you recognize which products should not be promoted and what kind of activities are considered to be promotion.

UK law

In the UK, marketing of breast milk substitutes is regulated by law through the Infant Formula and Follow on Formula Regulations 2007. This is meant to restrict advertising of formula so as not to discourage breastfeeding. However, it is not as robust as the code because it allows marketing of follow-on formula. This means that companies can advertise their logos on television, in magazines and on social media, and because the logos are the same for both standard formula and follow-on formula, this has the end result of publicizing both (Entwistle 2013).

UNICEF Baby Friendly Initiative

The Baby Friendly Initiative is a worldwide programme that started in 1992 to encourage maternity hospitals to practice in accordance with the code and implement the 10 steps to successful breastfeeding. In 1998 this was extended to community healthcare provision through introduction of the seven-point plan. The best practice standards set out in these 10 steps and the seven-point plan are seen as the minimum standard and are recommended in the postnatal NICE guideline (NICE 2006). In 2012, following extensive consultation, new standards were launched. These incorporate the 10 steps and seven-point plan but update and expand them to incorporate recent evidence. In these new standards, there is increased focus on relationship building between parents and their babies, and at Stage 3 the standards apply separately to maternity services, neonatal units, health visiting/public health nursing services and early years settings such as children's centres. A document collating high-quality evidence that underpins these standards has been produced and can be downloaded from the UNICEF Baby Friendly website (Entwistle 2013).

Activity

Access the current standards for healthcare facilities and/or the learning outcomes for universities at https://www.unicef.org.uk/babyfriendly/baby-friendly-resources/guidance-for-health-professionals/implementing-the-baby-friendly-standards/. Consider how this might affect your practice. Download 'The evidence and rationale for the UNICEF UK Baby Friendly Initiative Standards' at https://www.unicef.org.uk/babyfriendly/baby-friendly-resources/advocacy/the-evidence-and-rationale-for-the-unicef-uk-baby-friendly-initiative-standards/ and read Chapter 4 that sets out the evidence relating to parents' experiences.

REFLECTION ON THE TRIGGER SCENARIO

Look back at the trigger scenario.

> Sadie is breastfeeding her baby, Tom. She has recently had a visit from her mother who has undermined her confidence by telling her that she is 'probably not feeding Tom enough or that her milk is not strong enough' because he is feeding often. Sadie is now not sure whether to carry on breastfeeding – after all, she and her three brothers are all very healthy and they were all fed formula. She looks down at baby Tom who is lying in her arms gazing up at her face and says 'I just want you to grow, be strong, healthy and happy'. Sadie decides she will ask the community midwife when she visits later in the day.

Sadie's experience is not uncommon. If you were the community midwife visiting Sadie that day, what information would you give her? Are there any strategies she might use to cope with potentially unhelpful comments from her mother? Might she benefit from meeting with other breastfeeding mothers? What information might she need about formula feeding?

The scenario highlights that a new mother's confidence in her ability to breastfeed may be easily undermined. When a new mother arrives home from hospital with her new baby, she may feel particularly vulnerable. However, if the community midwife takes time to listen to Sadie's concerns, she may be able to boost her self-confidence and support her to breastfeed her baby. Now that you are familiar with some of the unique components of breast milk and the risks of formula feeding, you should have an insight into how the scenario relates to the evidence. The jigsaw model will now be used to explore the trigger scenario in more depth.

Effective communication

If Sadie asks the community midwife about formula feeding and believes it to be as good as breastfeeding, a careful exploration of this will need to take place. The midwife must give accurate information about the differences between feeding formula and breastfeeding whilst acknowledging and taking account of Sadie's beliefs and understanding. To do this, it will be essential for the community midwife to listen carefully to Sadie, and she may use communication techniques such as reflecting back to show that she is listening. Questions that arise from the scenario might include: Would this conversation be easier for both Sadie and the community midwife if they already had an established relationship? How can the midwife give accurate information about formula feeding without making Sadie feel uncomfortable? Would it be helpful for the community midwife to speak to Sadie's mother?

Woman-centred care

Any conversation about mode of feeding should take into account the woman's individual circumstances and should address her concerns. It appears from the scenario that Sadie had chosen to breastfeed and was happy with this decision until her mother came to visit. As discussed in Chapter 6, women's choices can be reinforced or constrained by people in their family or social network. For example, if a mother's own mother has breastfed, she is more likely to continue breastfeeding for longer. Questions that arise from the scenario might include: What kinds of questions might the community midwife ask Sadie? How might she use what Sadie says to provide further information about infant feeding? Would it be helpful to explore Sadie's partner's beliefs about infant feeding?

Using best evidence

Biological studies continue to contribute to the understanding of the complex actions and interactions of the living components of breast milk, and many epidemiological studies highlight associations between breastfeeding and a wide range of positive outcomes. However, knowledge of these factors must be communicated carefully to women and their families. Often, women are aware that 'breast is best' and reinforcing this can leave them feeling that they are 'bad mothers' if they choose to feed their baby formula (Murphy 1999). Questions that arise from the scenario might include: What kind of support has been shown to be most helpful for mothers like Sadie? What does Sadie know about the components of formula? If Sadie chooses to change to formula feeding, does she know how to sterilize bottles and make up a feed? At what point would it be appropriate for the community midwife to ensure Sadie knows these things but without undermining her confidence in her ability to breastfeed even more?

Professional and legal issues

Midwives should listen to people in their care and 'respond to their preferences and concerns' (NMC 2015:4). This is especially relevant to the choices mothers may make in relation to infant feeding. Sadie, like many women, may be constrained in her choice to breastfeed by the culture and environment in which she lives. If women choose to formula feed, it is important that they feel well supported. Questions that arise from the scenario might include: How might the community midwife respond to Sadie's concerns? What resources might the community midwife give to Sadie after their conversation? How does the community midwife ensure that her knowledge about breastfeeding and formula feeding is up to date? How might the conversation be documented?

Team working

The community midwife is continuing the care that was provided for Sadie in the hospital, and she is doing this working in partnership with Sadie and her family. There will be others in the primary healthcare team and local community that the midwife may also liaise with. Questions that arise from the scenario might include: Are there local infant feeding supporters in the area where Sadie lives? If Sadie chose to continue breastfeeding but encountered a challenge during the night and was concerned, whom would she contact? When will the community midwife visit Sadie next?

Clinical dexterity

The midwife will need knowledge of a range of infant feeding practices including an in-depth knowledge of why breastfeeding is the healthiest option for babies and the risks of formula feeding. When a midwife has in-depth knowledge of this, she will find it easier to communicate accurate information in response to each woman's needs. The most important skill in this scenario will be sensitive communication, but if Sadie chooses to continue to breastfeed then skilful breastfeeding support may also be needed. If at some stage she chooses to bottle feed, then clear information and instructions will be essential to ensure she knows how. Questions that arise from the scenario might include: If all Sadie needed was some reassurance to boost her confidence and feel she can continue to breastfeed, what would the midwife do? If Sadie had decided to give formula, would the midwife simply tell Sadie how to make up a feed or would she show her what to do? Would the midwife leave any written information about this? Might a conversation about mixed feeding be helpful?

Models of care

A model of care that provides continuity is likely to be most helpful to Sadie in this situation. If she already knows the community midwife, there may already be a relationship of trust, and this is likely to make potentially difficult conversations easier. Questions that arise from the scenario might include: At what point did Sadie have her first conversation about infant feeding with the midwife? How might the community midwife have built up a trusting relationship? When did Sadie decide she wanted to breastfeed?

Safe environment

A breastfed baby is more likely to remain safe due to the protective factors within breast milk. However, if Sadie chooses to give formula to her baby then to keep her baby safe, she will need to know that she should sterilize all equipment, that powdered formula is not sterile and that she should make up a feed each time her baby needs one. Questions that arise from the scenario might include: How is a breastfed baby protected from bacteria that the mother and baby are exposed to? There is a range of other factors that might impact on the safety of a bottle feeding infant; what are these factors? What would Sadie need to know about bottle feeding her baby?

Promotes health

There is no doubt that breastfeeding is the healthiest option for babies worldwide, as demonstrated in a recent review of the evidence (Victora et al 2016). These health effects last into adulthood and future generations. Midwives should ensure they support women who have made the choice to breastfeed but also to respect and support the decisions of those women who do not. Questions that arise from the scenario might include: Do you think Sadie is aware of the advantages of breastfeeding? Which of these might be most important to her? What is the World Health Organization's recommendation for optimal infant feeding?

Further scenarios

The following scenarios enable you to consider how specific situations influence the care the midwife provides. Use the jigsaw model to explore the issues raised in each situation.

SCENARIO 1

Lucy had her first baby, Kylie, yesterday, and she is preparing to go home from the midwife-led unit where she gave birth. Lucy has always intended to feed Kylie by bottle because she feels very sensitive about the size of her breasts. She does not feel able to breastfeed for this reason. Lucy does not know how to make up a formula feed and has just asked the midwife, Stacey, if she can show her how to do this.

Practice point

Many women do not make up formula feeds as recommended. It is therefore crucial that they are given clear information about how to sterilize bottles and make up feeds so that they fully understand the importance of this. It is also important to discuss ways that mothers who have chosen to formula feed can maximize opportunities to build a close and loving relationship with their baby.

Further points specific to Scenario 1 include:

1. When might a conversation about infant feeding have taken place during antenatal care and would it necessarily have been helpful to find out how Lucy intended to feed at that point?

2. Did Lucy have time skin-to-skin with her baby after birth? Some women change their mind about feeding if their baby crawls to the breast after birth, but they may not feel able to change their mind if they have been encouraged to state their decision.

3. Once Lucy has chosen that she want to bottle feed, how will she be supported to do this?

4. Will Lucy be shown how to make up a feed?

5. What written resources could Lucy be given?

SCENARIO 2

Cathy had her baby 5 days ago and is talking to the community midwife, Jayne, about feeding. Cathy has been breastfeeding her baby, Saskia, since birth but is finding frequent feeding a challenge. Cathy has just explained to Jayne that she is considering feeding Saskia both breast and bottle 'because bottle feeding is just as good as breastfeeding really, isn't it?'

Practice point

Clear, sensitive evidence-based conversations about the difference between breastfeeding and formula feeding are important in situations like Cathy's. The midwife will need to ensure that Cathy has this information but also that she understands the effect that replacing a breastfeed with a formula feed will have on her milk supply.

Further points specific to Scenario 2 include:

1. What might Jayne's response be and how can she ensure that Cathy makes an informed choice?

2. Could Jayne explore what Cathy knows about the effects of formula feeding on the baby's gut?

3. Women often think that a baby will sleep more if given formula feeds. This may sometimes be the case, but why is this?

4. There are many books available that unhelpfully advocate routines and regular feeding of young babies. Might it be useful to ask Cathy what she has read about infant feeding?

5. Sometimes women decide to introduce a formula feed to enable their partner to feed the baby. If this were part of the decision-making process for Cathy, what would she need to know about the effect on her supply of breast milk?

Conclusion

Midwives have a responsibility to give women accurate evidence-based information about both breastfeeding and formula feeding, and this should include a discussion about the risks of formula feeding. If a woman decides she wishes to formula feed, she should be fully supported and this should include showing her how to make up feeds correctly and giving information about different types of formula feeds, taking care not to contravene the code.

Resources

Crawley, H. & Westland, S. *Infant milks in the UK: A practical guide for health professionals.* Available at: http://www.firststepsnutrition.org/newpages/infants/infant_feeding_infant_milks_UK.html.

First Steps Nutrition. Available at: http://www.firststepsnutrition.org/newpages/infants/infant_feeding_infant_milks_UK.html.

The Infant Formula and Follow-on Formula (England) Regulations 2007. Available at: http://www.legislation.gov.uk/uksi/2007/3521/contents/made.

NHS guide to bottle feeding 2011. Available at: http://www.pat.nhs.uk/downloads/patient-information-leaflets/maternity/after-birth/Guide%20to%20bottle%20feeding.pdf.

The International Code of Marketing of Breast-Milk Substitutes. Available at: http://www.who.int/nutrition/publications/infantfeeding/9241541601/en/.

UNICEF Guide to bottle feeding. Available at: http://www.unicef.org.uk/Documents/Baby_Friendly/Leaflets/guide_to_bottle_feeding.pdf.

References

Aaltonen, J., Ojala, T., Laitinen, K., et al., 2011. Impact of maternal diet during pregnancy and breastfeeding on infant metabolic programming: a prospective randomized controlled study. Eur. J. Clin. Nutr. 65, 10–19.

Azad, M.B., Konya, T., Persaud, R.R., et al., 2016. Impact of maternal intrapartum antibiotics, method of birth and breastfeeding on gut microbiota during the first year of life: a prospective cohort study. BJOG 123, 983–993.

Bolling, K., Grant, C., Hamlyn, B., Thornton, A., 2007. Infant feeding survey 2005. London: The Information Centre.

Cabrera-Rubio, R., Collado, M.C., Laitinen, K., et al., 2012. The human milk microbiome changes over lactation and is shaped by maternal weight and mode of delivery. Am. J. Clin. Nutr. 96, 544.

Crawley, H., Westland, S., 2016. Infant milks in the UK: A practical guide for health professionals. London: First Steps Nutrition Trust.

Entwistle, F.M., 2013. The evidence and rationale for the UNICEF UK Baby Friendly Initiative standards. London: UNICEF UK.

Hoddinott, P., Tappin, D., Wright, C., 2008. Breast feeding. BMJ 336, 881–887.

Ip, S., Chung, M., Raman, G., et al., 2009. A summary of the Agency for Healthcare Research and Quality's evidence report on breastfeeding in developed countries. Breastfeed. Med. 4 (s1), S-17–S-30.

Jiménez, E., Marín, M.L., Martín, R., et al., 2008. Is meconium from healthy newborns actually sterile? Res. Microbiol. 159, 187–193.

McAndrew, F., Thompson, J., Fellows, L., et al., 2012. Infant Feeding Survey 2010. London: Health and Social Care Information Centre.

Morelli, L., 2008. Postnatal development of intestinal microflora as influenced by infant nutrition. J. Nutr. 138, 1791S–1795S.

Murphy, E., 1999. 'Breast is best': Infant feeding decisions and maternal deviance. Sociol Health Illn 21, 187–208.

Neu, J., 2016. The microbiome during pregnancy and early postnatal life. Semin. Fetal Neonatal Med. 21, 373–379.

NICE, 2006. Routine postnatal care of women and their babies. London: NICE.

NMC, 2015. The code: professional standards of practice and behaviour for nurses and midwives. London: Nursing and Midwifery Council. Available at: https://www.nmc.org.uk/globalassets/sitedocuments/nmc-publications/nmc-code.pdf.

Palmer, G., 2009. The Politics of Breastfeeding: When Breasts Are Bad for Business. Pinter and Martin, London.

Penders, J., Thijs, C., Vink, C., et al., 2006. Factors Influencing the composition of the intestinal microbiota in early infancy. Pediatrics 118, 511–521.

Quigley, M.A., Kelly, Y.J., Sacker, A., 2007. Breastfeeding and hospitalization for diarrheal and respiratory infection in the United Kingdom Millennium Cohort Study. Pediatrics 119, e837–e842.

UNICEF Baby Friendly Initiative UK & Department of Health, 2013. Guide to bottle feeding: how to prepare infant formula and sterilise feeding equipment to minimise the risks to your baby. London: Crown.

UNICEF Baby Friendly UK & First Steps Nutrition Trust, 2016. Guide for parents who are formula feeding. London: UNICEF Baby Friendly.

Victora, C.G., Bahl, R., Barros, A.J.D., et al., 2016. Breastfeeding in the 21st century: epidemiology, mechanisms, and lifelong effect. Lancet 387, 475–490.

Walker, M., 2013. Breastfeeding Management for the Clinician: Using the Evidence, fourth ed. Jones and Bartlett, London.

WHO Collaborative Study Team on the Role of Breastfeeding on the Prevention of Infant Mortality, 2000. Effect of breastfeeding on infant and child mortality due to infectious diseases in less developed countries: a pooled analysis. Lancet 355, 451–455.

World Health Organisation, 1981. International Code of Marketing of Breast-Milk Substitutes. Geneva: World Health Organisation.

World Health Organisation, 2003. Global strategy for infant and young child feeding. Geneva: World Health Organisation.

CHAPTER 10

Managing common maternal-related breastfeeding challenges

TRIGGER SCENARIO

Gail has been breastfeeding baby Carla for a week now since her birth. A few days after she came home from the hospital, she had experienced some soreness whilst feeding, and her nipples had become cracked. The community midwife watched Carla breastfeed and made some suggestions to Gail to help her to position Carla differently. This helped and Gail's nipples have since been healing well, but today she is feeling unwell with flu-like symptoms and has noticed a reddened area on the outer aspect of her left breast.

Introduction

In the UK, around 30% of mothers experience breastfeeding challenges in the early weeks and only around a quarter are still exclusively breastfeeding when their baby is 6 weeks old (McAndrew et al 2012). Midwives have a responsibility to provide support to breastfeeding women (NICE 2006), and the most recent infant feeding survey shows that women who receive help or support are more likely to continue breastfeeding (McAndrew et al 2012). The challenges most commonly experienced by women in the first 2 weeks of breastfeeding include the baby finding it difficult to latch onto the breast and/or breast discomfort or painful nipples (McAndrew et al 2012). Reasons why a baby may be sleepy or not attach well at the breast have been discussed in Chapters 7 and 8. Many of the maternal-related challenges can be resolved if identified early and attention given to improving positioning and attachment enabling women to continue to breastfeed.

UNICEF Baby Friendly Maternity standards

The following are the maternity standards that are most relevant to this chapter:
- Support all mothers and babies to initiate a close relationship and feeding soon after birth
- Enable mothers to get breastfeeding off to a good start

Sore and painful nipples

Many women experience some nipple tenderness in the first few days as they and their baby learn the skill of breastfeeding, but this should not last long and should not be painful. Sore nipples are most likely to occur if the baby is not positioned and/or attached well at the breast. As discussed in Chapter 5, attachment is how the baby takes the breast into her mouth to enable her to feed and positioning is how the mother holds her baby to enable her to attach (UNICEF Baby Friendly Initiative UK 2014). If a baby has taken a large mouthful of breast tissue into her mouth, then the mother's nipple will be protected at the back of the mouth against the soft palate rather than rubbing against the hard palate. When a baby releases the breast, if the nipple is misshaped, this means the baby could be better attached or positioned more optimally.

Nipple pain and trauma can cause a mother to become anxious and can affect her relationship with her baby (McClellan et al 2012). It can lead to a tendency to feed less often; also the release of oxytocin may be inhibited so that milk may not flow as easily which can compound the problem (Walker 2013). If a mother is experiencing sore and/or traumatized nipples, the midwife should take a lactation history, observe a complete breastfeed to assess the baby's position and attachment and sucking pattern and assess the baby to exclude anomalies such as tongue-tie. If a mother has flat or inverted nipples, she should be reassured that the baby will be able to breastfeed as babies feed from the breast rather than the nipple.

Nipple pain is often worst around 3 days after birth (Walker 2013). A Cochrane review that has investigated various interventions that might be helpful for sore nipples found that nothing or expressed breast milk rubbed on the mother's nipples appeared to be equally or more effective than the application of ointments such as lanolin. Although the quality of the included studies was good, overall there was generally a paucity of good quality evidence for the primary outcome of nipple pain (Dennis et al 2014). This review also found that, for most women, nipple pain was considerably reduced by 10 days after birth which may be helpful for women to know, to encourage continuation of exclusive breastfeeding (Dennis et al 2014).

Persistent nipple pain may be associated with abnormal sucking and tongue movement as has been demonstrated in an ultrasound study (McClellan et al 2015). Nipple pain may be associated with other conditions of the breast such as engorgement or Thrush (discussed later) and can also be caused by other conditions such as eczema, dermatitis or Raynaud's disease (Anderson et al 2004; Morino & Winn 2007). Nipple trauma can provide a portal for organisms to enter the breast causing either bacterial or fungal infection.

Activity

Consider a variety of different ways of explaining to mothers how to position and attach their baby onto the breast. Mothers learn in different ways, so it is useful to have a range of resources to help with this. The graphic of a baby attaching on the breast may be useful for some mothers and can be found at https://www.bestbeginnings.org.uk/graphic-of-a-baby-attaching-on-the-breast/067348cf-7dd7-46cb-8f8b-9ae5ddaad028. Read some articles about Raynaud's disease (e.g. Anderson et al 2004). Ensure you can recognize the symptoms of and treatment for Raynaud's disease; a photograph of a breast affected by this is available in Heller et al (2012).

Engorgement

A mother's breasts may be very full when the milk 'comes in' between the third and sixth day after giving birth, and this is usually resolved easily if the baby is feeding effectively at the breast. It is important for the midwife to be able to distinguish between full breasts, which are firm and full often with a marbled appearance, and engorged breasts that are painfully full, shiny and oedematous with reddened areas (World Health Organization 2000). If a woman's breasts are engorged, the milk does not flow well because the breasts are not only full of milk but also tissue fluid and venous, and lymphatic drainage are obstructed (UNICEF Baby Friendly Initiative UK 2014). The nipple sometimes becomes flattened and the surrounding areola becomes much firmer, making it more difficult for the baby to attach and feed well, and this can lead to damaged nipples.

Engorgement can be prevented by ensuring milk is removed regularly and efficiently by making sure the baby is fully attached to the breast, positioned optimally and is feeding often. If observed, engorgement needs to be treated quickly otherwise a woman's milk supply may diminish and stasis of milk may result in blocked ducts and mastitis. When the breasts are full, the milk supply will be reduced by the presence of feedback inhibitor of lactation (FIL) – a whey protein which regulates milk production within each breast. If the baby is finding it difficult to attach to an engorged breast, gentle hand expression may be required to soften the breast tissue. If the breasts are still full after the baby has fed, further expression may be needed. Warmth on the breasts may help the milk to flow more easily, and the mother may require analgesia such as paracetamol or ibuprofen.

A range of treatments have been suggested to relieve engorgement, such as heat therapy, cold therapy, chilled cabbage leaves, acupuncture, acupressure, preotease complex and gua-sha (scraping therapy); however, the effectiveness of these is not certain. A Cochrane review found only small studies and was inconclusive but suggests 'hot/cold packs, gua-sha (scraping therapy), acupuncture, cabbage leaves and proteolytic enzymes may be promising' (Mangesi & Zakarija-Grkovic 2016:2).

Activity

If there is a build-up of breast milk in the breast, what is present that causes a reduction in milk supply? Access the Internet and find a video clip explaining hand expression that you think would be useful for women to watch.

Mastitis

Mastitis is an inflammatory response within the breast which is usually caused by stasis of milk. When not adequately drained from the breast, the milk collects in the alveoli causing increased pressure and distension which can often be felt as a tender, palpable lump. When this occurs, components of the milk are forced through the cell walls into the capillaries or tissue, and these trigger an immune response (Deshpande 2007). Mastitis can happen at any point during lactation but most occur in the first

12 weeks postpartum, most commonly in the second and third week (World Health Organization 2000).

If a breastfeeding mother has flu-like symptoms, mastitis should always be suspected as this can be the first sign (Noonan 2010). A mother with mastitis may complain of general aches and pains, headache and chills and fever, and a red, swollen area of the breast may be visible (Wambach 2016). To diagnose mastitis, it is important to take a breastfeeding history from the mother to identify any likely causal factors (Pollard 2012). Any factor that leads to the breast not being fully drained can predispose to mastitis. Commonly, this can be poor positioning and attachment leading to inefficient milk transfer, but can also be factors such as the baby having limited time at the breast, missed feeds through, for example, supplementary bottle feeds or use of a dummy or the baby having a short frenulum (tongue-tie). Sore and cracked nipples can lead a mother to delay feeding and can also mean that bacteria can enter the breast more easily. If there has been pressure on the breast for any length of time, for example, from a tight bra or a mother holding her breast whilst feeding, the milk flow can be reduced (Wambach 2016). A Cochrane review has assessed the effectiveness of a range of factors with potential to prevent mastitis, such as breastfeeding education, taking antibiotic medication, topical ointments and anti-secretory factor cereal, and none were found to have any effect (Crepinsek et al 2012).

When a mother has mastitis, it is important to ensure the baby feeds as much as possible and that breast drainage is achieved (UNICEF Baby Friendly Initiative UK 2014). It may be helpful for the mother to feed from the affected breast first to ensure effective removal of as much milk as possible from that breast. It is also important to observe a breastfeed and ensure good positioning and attachment. A warm compress may be helpful to help the milk flow. If the baby does not feed well on the affected breast, then the milk should be expressed. Sometimes babies are reluctant to feed; possibly due to the milk tasting more salty than usual because the inflammatory response causes the junctions between the cells in the alveoli to open allowing sodium and immunoproteins to pass through (World Health Organization 2000). This is usually temporary, lasting about a week.

Whether the mastitis is or is not due to infection, mothers are likely to feel relief from anti-inflammatory medication. Non-steroidal anti-inflammatory medication such as ibuprofen 400 mg three times a day can be given to reduce the inflammation and pain as long as the mother does not suffer from asthma or stomach ulcers (The Breastfeeding Network 2015). Paracetamol 1 g four times a day may also be given to relieve pain and reduce pyrexia, but aspirin should not be taken by breastfeeding women (The Breastfeeding Network 2015). If there is no improvement seen, infection may be present and antibiotics may be the next line of treatment.

A Cochrane review has investigated the effectiveness of antibiotic therapy to relieve the symptoms of mastitis in breastfeeding women; however, insufficient evidence was found to reach a conclusion and further high-quality research was recommended (Jahanfar et al 2013). It is generally recommended that if the mother does not feel any improvements within 12 to 24 hours by increasing feeding and breast drainage and taking anti-inflammatory medication, then she should contact her general practitioner as this is indicative of the need for antibiotics. She will also need support; a mother who has mastitis feels unwell and often becomes emotional and may feel like discontinuing breastfeeding, which would compound the situation.

Activity

Mastitis often starts with a blocked milk duct. What might you say to a woman to help to prevent this? When would be the best time to educate women about the possibility of milk ducts becoming blocked? Read about white spot on the nipple. What would you advise a woman with this to do?

Perceived insufficient milk supply

For women who have started breastfeeding, the perception that they do not have enough milk for their baby is a common concern and can lead women to stop breastfeeding or not to breastfeed exclusively (Andrews et al 2007; Gatti 2008). Actual insufficient milk supply is rare. Sometimes mothers can perceive that they have insufficient milk in the first 24 to 48 hours after birth if they are not prepared for the small quantities of colostrum needed by the baby at this stage of feeding (Walker 2013). The use of 'belly balls' to visually convey the size of the baby's stomach can be helpful to allay these fears. Perceptions of low supply can be reinforced if women attempt to express and this only yields a few drops of colostrum (Walker 2013). However, this may be due to anxiety affecting oxytocin and the 'let down' of milk rather than an actual problem with supply, and this is usually only temporary.

The inability to directly observe the amount of milk their baby is taking is one of the underlying concerns for women when they are worried about their milk supply, and this is exacerbated when the baby is not settling well after feeds (Marshall et al 2007). Once breastfeeding is established, many women draw on indirect signs that their baby is feeding well. These include things like softer breasts after feeds, their baby having wet and dirty nappies and the baby gaining weight. However, women are vulnerable to negative comments from members of their family and close social networks (as discussed in Chapter 6).

A crying and unsettled baby is one of the most common reasons women think they do not have enough milk. If mothers perceive this as hunger, then they may decide to introduce a formula feed. This then reduces the baby's suckling at the breast and ultimately lower prolactin production leads to an actual reduction in milk supply. Full breasts from a missed breastfeed and the presence of FIL within the breast milk will also reduce milk supply. If, however, mothers are supported when their baby is unsettled and a supporter observes a feed to ensure the baby is feeding effectively, supports the mother emotionally and ensures the mother understands that more frequent feeding will mean she produces more breast milk, this may mean the mother is reassured. It is important to rule out sucking problems such as tongue-tie (discussed in Chapter 8). Other techniques that the mother may find helpful include: frequent feeding, close contact with the baby including skin-to-skin contact, gentle breast massage and relaxation techniques.

Thrush (candida albicans)

Thrush causes an agonizing pain in both breasts after feeds and rarely occurs in the first 6 weeks after birth (Jones 2014). It is important that thrush is correctly diagnosed to avoid unnecessary treatment of mother and baby (Jones & Breward 2010) as nipple and/or breast pain is much more likely to be due to the need to improve positioning and attachment. Signs and symptoms of nipple thrush include: sudden onset of painful feeding after experiencing pain-free feeding, nipples redder than normal and unusually sensitive, signs of fungal infection in the baby and the baby may be unsettle or 'fussy' during feeding. It is always important to watch a baby feed and to rule out other possible reasons for breast pain, such as tongue-tie, Raynaud's syndrome or allergies to ointments or breast pads that may cause nipples to flake and itch (Jones & Breward 2010).

If thrush is suspected, then swabs should be taken from the mother's nipples and the baby's mouth to confirm this (Jones 2014). If thrush is identified, treatment should be started for both mother and baby. Thrush can be just on the nipple and this should be treated with topical application of antifungal cream (such as Miconazole 2%) applied sparingly to the nipples after every feed. The baby should be treated with oral antifungal gel at the same time. If symptoms persist, then further treatment might be necessary. Thrush can infect the milk ducts in the mother's breast, and this would require systemic treatment if topical treatment is not effective but only once swabs have been taken.

Activity

Read the leaflet 'Thrush and breastfeeding' available on The Breastfeeding Network website. Look up the drugs that are likely to be used to treat thrush in the British National Formulary.

REFLECTION ON THE TRIGGER SCENARIO

Look back at the trigger scenario.

> Gail has been breastfeeding baby Carla for a week now since her birth. A few days after she came home from the hospital, she had experienced some soreness whilst feeding, and her nipples had become cracked. The community midwife watched Carla breastfeed and made some suggestions to Gail to help her to position Carla differently. This helped and Gail's nipples have since been healing well, but today she is feeling unwell with flu-like symptoms and has noticed a reddened area on the outer aspect of her left breast.

Gail has received support from the community midwife to help her to breastfeed more effectively and reduce the soreness she experienced in the first few days. However, she is now feeling unwell. What is the most likely cause of her flu-like symptoms? What is the initial treatment for this? What information will she require about feeding? What might you suggest to help her feel better?

The jigsaw model will now be used to explore the trigger scenario in more depth.

Effective communication

The midwife should take time to obtain an accurate history from Gail to enable her to diagnose the problem. Once she has identified this, she will need to communicate carefully with Gail to encourage her to continue breastfeeding. When mothers are feeling unwell, they may become demotivated. But encouragement to continue feeding often will ultimately help Gail to recover. Questions that arise from the scenario might include: Why would it be important for the midwife to listen to Gail's concerns? What suggestions might the midwife make? How might the midwife attend to Gail's emotional wellbeing as well as her physical needs? If anyone is at home supporting Gail, what might the midwife say to them?

Woman-centred care

Most women want help and support that is specific for their needs at that time, rather than abstract, more generalized information that could be provided to anyone. Questions that arise from the scenario might include: How would the midwife ensure that information and support provided to Gail was specific to her needs? The midwife has watched Carla feed; what in particular would she have been assessing? What might the midwife suggest that could alleviate Gail's symptoms most quickly? When would the midwife contact or visit Gail next? What would the midwife suggest if Gail's symptoms do not improve in the next 24 hours?

Using best evidence

Evidence for effective factors that may prevent mastitis is lacking (Crepinsek et al 2012) as is evidence for the effectiveness of treatment with antibiotics (Jahanfar et al 2009). Larger, high-quality research studies are needed to inform clinical practice in relation to mastitis. Questions that arise from the scenario might include: What may have led to mastitis in Gail's case? What factors might the midwife have assessed in relation to the baby's ability to suck? What is happening at the cellular level to cause inflammation when a woman has mastitis? Why might the baby be reluctant to feed?

Professional and legal issues

Midwives must ensure that they take account of and assess mothers' physical, social and psychological needs and respond to these (NMC 2015). In a situation such as the one in this scenario, this is essential. Taking account of Gail's psychological needs, such as providing reassurance and emotional support within the context of her family and social situation, is as important as attending to her physical needs. Questions that arise from the scenario might include: How might the midwife find out about sources of support within Gail's social network? How might the midwife involve Gail's partner? How might this visit have been documented?

Team working

The community midwife works as part of the multi-disciplinary team in primary care. This will include Gail's general practitioner if her symptoms do not improve within 12 to 24 hours. It is important that other members of the team are adequately trained to support breastfeeding women and breastfed babies. Questions that arise from the scenario might include:

What medication would the midwife suggest Gail should take? Would the pharmacist give any advice? What would the midwife advise Gail to do if her symptoms did not start to improve within a few hours? If another member of the team suggested that Gail should not feed on the affected side, how should the midwife respond?

Clinical dexterity

The midwife will have provided care earlier when Gail's nipples became sore. This will have involved watching Carla feed and ensuring good attachment. Recognition of good attachment and effective feeding is a key skill required when supporting breastfeeding women. Questions that arise from the scenario might include: If Carla is well attached to the breast, what key features would the midwife observe? What are the principles of good positioning for breastfeeding? What sucking pattern would you expect to see if Carla was feeding effectively? Would the midwife suggest Gail to keep Carla near her? If so, why?

Models of care

The midwife may work within a model of care that means she will be able to visit Gail the next day, but this cannot always happen. Sometimes, days off or holidays mean that another member of the team will provide care. If this were to be the case, clear and accurate communication would be required to ensure Gail receives the care she needs. Questions that arise from the scenario might include: What would be the key factors to communicate if another midwife was to visit Gail? Would Gail have met that midwife before? Who has overall responsibility for Gail's care? Who would Gail contact if she was concerned about something?

Safe environment

The midwife has identified that the cause of Gail's illness is mastitis. If mastitis is not identified, it can lead to a breast abscess and could even lead to generalized sepsis. Therefore prompt management and optimal treatment of the condition is essential to maintain Gail's safety.

Questions that arise from the scenario might include: What is the most important aspect of the initial management of mastitis? What drugs would initially be suggested that would help to maintain the flow of breast milk? What would be suggested if the initial management had little effect?

Promotes health

Good management of a condition such as mastitis can resolve the situation quickly and will be more likely to ensure the mother feels able to continue to breastfeed. This is therefore health promoting at the time for the woman, as she will recover more quickly. Ultimately, continued breastfeeding will ensure the health of the baby is optimal, both at the time by preventing conditions such as gastroenteritis and later in life through reducing the risk of conditions such as overweight and diabetes (Victora et al 2016). Questions that arise from the scenario might include: Did the midwife tell Gail what to expect if the condition worsened? What would the midwife say if Gail was concerned about the baby feeding on the affected breast?

Further scenarios

The following scenarios enable you to consider how specific situations influence the care the midwife provides. Use the jigsaw model to explore the issues raised in each situation.

SCENARIO 1

Sophie is the community midwife who has just arrived at Helen's home. She finds Helen pacing up and down with baby George, who is unsettled and fractious. Helen says to Sophie 'I just don't think he is getting enough milk'.

Practice point

An unsettled baby who cries frequently is often the cause of women's concern about milk supply. This can be reinforced by comments from family members or others in the mother's social network.

Further points specific to Scenario 1 include:
1. What might Sophie say to Helen?
2. What might she do during the visit?
3. What conditions in the baby might Sophie want to observe for and rule out?
4. Might Sophie suggest skin-to-skin contact with George and a laid-back position for breastfeeding?
5. Why might this be helpful?

SCENARIO 2

Sally had her baby, Anna, 4 days ago. She has telephoned the community midwife because she is not able to breastfeed Anna. Her breasts are very full and tender, and the skin on her breasts is tense and shiny. Sally explains all of this to the community midwife with tears rolling down her cheeks.

> **Practice point**
>
> In situations such as the one in this scenario, it is important to be able to distinguish between breasts that are full of milk and breasts that are engorged.

Further points specific to Scenario 2 include:

1. What is the likely physiological cause of the tenderness in Sally's breasts?
2. Would the midwife visit Sally?
3. What needs to happen urgently to preserve Sally's milk supply and why?
4. Why might the breast milk not flow easily?
5. What would the midwife suggest that Sally should do?

Conclusion

Maternal-related breastfeeding challenges are relatively common and distressing for mothers. If such challenges are not recognized and resolved quickly, mothers are likely to stop breastfeeding. Midwives should be alert to the signs and symptoms of these conditions as they have an important role to play in correctly diagnosing them and offering relevant evidence-based information to enable resolution and continued breastfeeding.

References

Anderson, J.E., Held, N., Wright, K., 2004. Raynaud's phenomenon of the nipple: a treatable cause of painful breastfeeding. Pediatrics 113, e360–e364.

Andrews, J.I., Fleener, D.K., Messer, S.A., et al., 2007. The yeast connection: is Candida linked to breastfeeding associated pain? Am. J. Obstet. Gynecol. 197, 424.e1–424.e4.

Crepinsek, M.A., Crowe, L., Michener, K., Smart, N.A., 2012. Interventions for preventing mastitis after childbirth. Cochrane Database Syst. Rev. (10), Art. No.: CD007239, doi:10.1002/14651858.CD007239.pub3.

Dennis, C.-L., Jackson, K., Watson, J., 2014. Interventions for treating painful nipples among breastfeeding women. Cochrane Database Syst. Rev. (12), Art. No.CD007366, doi:10.1002/14651858.CD007366.pub2.

Deshpande, W., 2007. Mastitis. Community Pract. 80, 44–45.

Gatti, L., 2008. Maternal perceptions of insufficient milk supply in breastfeeding. J. Nurs. Scholarsh. 40, 355–363.

Heller, M.M., Fullerton-Stone, H., Murase, J.E., 2012. Caring for new mothers: diagnosis, management and treatment of nipple dermatitis in breastfeeding mothers. Int. J. Dermatol. 51, 1149–1161.

Jahanfar, S., Ng, C., Teng, C., 2009. Antibiotics for mastitis in breastfeeding women. Cochrane Database Syst. Rev. (1), Art. No.: CD005458, doi:10.1002/14651858. CD005458.pub2.

Jahanfar, S., Ng, C.J., Teng, C.L., 2013. Antibiotics for mastitis in breastfeeding women. Cochrane Database Syst. Rev. (2), Art. No. CD005458, doi:10.1002/14651858. CD005458.pub3.

Jones, W., 2014. Thrush and breastfeeding. Paisley: The Breasfeeding Network.

Jones, W., Breward, S., 2010. Thrush and breastfeeding. Community Pract. 83, 42–43.

Mangesi, L., Zakarija-Grkovic, I., 2016. Treatments for breast engorgement during lactation. Cochrane Database Syst. Rev. (6), CD006946.

Marshall, J.L., Godfrey, M., Renfrew, M.J., 2007. Being a 'good mother': managing breastfeeding and merging identities. Soc. Sci. Med. 65, 2147–2159.

McAndrew, F., Thompson, J., Fellows, L., et al., 2012, Infant Feeding Survey 2010. London: Health and Social Care Information Centre.

McClellan, H.L., Hepworth, A.R., Garbin, C.P., et al., 2012. Nipple pain during breastfeeding with or without visible trauma. J. Hum. Lact. 28, 511–521.

McClellan, H.L., Kent, J.C., Hepworth, A.R., et al., 2015. Persistent Nipple Pain in Breastfeeding Mothers Associated with Abnormal Infant Tongue Movement. Int. J. Environ. Res. Public Health 12, 10833–10845.

Morino, C., Winn, S.M., 2007. Raynaud's phenomenon of the nipples: an elusive diagnosis. J. Hum. Lact. 23, 191–193.

NICE, 2006. Routine postnatal care of women and their babies. London: NICE.

NMC, 2015. The code: Professional Standards of Practice and Behaviour for Nurses and Midwives. Nursing and Midwifery Council, London. Available at:: https://www.nmc.org.uk/globalassets/sitedocuments/nmc-publications/nmc-code.pdf.

Noonan, M., 2010. Lactational mastitis: recognition and breastfeeding support. BJM 18, 503–508.

Pollard, M., 2012. Evidence-Based Care for Breastfeeding mothers. Routledge, London.

The Breastfeeding Network, 2015. Mastitis and breastfeeding. Paisley: The Breastfeeding Network.

UNICEF Baby Friendly Initiative UK, 2014. The UNICEF UK Baby Friendly Initiative Train the Trainer. London: UNICEF Baby Friendly Initiative UK.

Victora, C.G., Bahl, R., Barros, A.J.D., et al., 2016. Breastfeeding in the 21st century: epidemiology, mechanisms, and lifelong effect. Lancet 387, 475–490.

Walker, M., 2013. Breastfeeding Management for the Clinician: Using the Evidence, fourth ed. Jones and Bartlett, London.

Wambach, K., 2016. Breast-related problems. In: Wambach, K., Riordan, J. (Eds.), Breastfeeding and Human Lactation, fifth ed. Jones and Bartlett, Burlington.

World Health Organization, 2000. Mastitis: Causes and Management. WHO, Geneva.

CHAPTER 11

Breastfeeding premature babies

TRIGGER SCENARIO

Baby Jack was born by caesarean section at 29 weeks' gestation as his mother, Lynne, had pregnancy-induced hypertension. Lynne enjoyed holding Jack against her skin immediately after birth in the operating theatre as he seemed calm and relaxed, although she was amazed at how small he seemed. Lynne is keen to start expressing breast milk for Jack and has asked the midwife what she should do.

Introduction

Having a premature baby can be a very frightening and traumatic experience for parents (Arnold 2010). They may be anxious and concerned about the health and possible survival of their infant and may spend long periods of time separated from them (Renfrew et al 2009). Mothers with a baby in the special care or neonatal intensive care unit (NICU) make the transition to motherhood in an unfamiliar and medicalized environment (Flacking et al 2006), and midwives caring for families of premature babies can do much to support them at this difficult time.

UNICEF Baby Friendly Maternity standards

The following are the maternity standards that are most relevant to this chapter:

- Support pregnant women to recognize the importance of breastfeeding and early relationships for the health and wellbeing of their baby
- Support all mothers and babies to initiate a close relationship and feeding soon after birth

---

Breast milk: 'a medicine' for premature babies

Breastfeeding is the optimal choice for all babies but being fed breast milk is especially important for premature infants. Specific biofactors such as immunoglobulin A (IgA), lactoferrin, lysozyme, growth factors and enzymes in human milk all contribute to decreased rates of infections in premature infants (Spatz 2016). There are many hazards of formula feeding affecting a broad range of outcomes for premature infants such as delayed brainstem maturation, poorer visual acuity and increased incidence of retinopathy of prematurity (e.g. Arnold 2010; Hurst & Meier 2010; Spatz 2016; Walker 2017). One of the most important issues to be aware of is that premature babies who are fed formula rather than human milk are around 6 to 10 times more likely to suffer from necrotizing enterocolitis (NEC) than babies who are fed either their mother's milk or donor human milk (Lucas & Cole 1990; McGuire & Anthony 2003). NEC is a disease of prematurity that causes significant mortality and morbidity. It is a condition that, if allowed to progress, can lead to ischaemia, gangrene and possibly perforation of the intestine (Arnold 2010). The risk of developing NEC is highest in infants born at earlier gestations. Lucas and Cole (1990) estimated that 400 cases and 100 deaths could be prevented each year if infants were fed human milk. A recent case control study has shown that very low birth weight babies who are not fed breast milk and/or are given parenteral nutrition are at higher risk of NEC and are recommended early enteral feeds of breast milk (Kimak et al 2015).

The gut of the premature infant is immature, and human milk contains components that help it to mature whereas formula does not (Walker 2017). Components in human milk are thought to promote closure of the junctions between cells in the lining of the gut and aid the digestion of proteins and carbohydrates. Whereas undigested casein in the gut from formula can attract neutrophils that provoke an inflammatory response and opening of the junctions between cells in the gut wall allowing invasion and damage to the premature infant's fragile gut (Walker 2017).

Extremely low birth weight infants fed human milk have also been shown to have better neurodevelopmental outcomes at 18 months of age than those not fed human milk in a dose-dependent relationship (Vohr et al 2006). This study of 1035 low birth weight infants showed that the more breast milk the infants ingested, the higher the mental developmental, psychomotor and behaviour scores (Vohr et al 2006). Analysis of data from the millennium cohort study has also demonstrated enhanced cognitive development at 5 years of age when an infant is breastfed at all, but the effects were greater when infants were breastfed for 4 months and if infants were premature (Quigley et al 2012). Premature infants have greater nutritional needs than full-term infants partly because of the immaturity of their digestive systems (Arnold 2010). The composition of milk from mothers of premature infants differs from that of mothers of term babies; it is higher in many nutrients for about the first 2 to 4 weeks (Arnold 2010). For all these reasons, premature babies should be fed human milk unless medically contra-indicated.

Parents of premature infants have a right to factual information about the effects that human milk feeding will have so that their feeding decisions can be based on current evidence. Most mothers, even if they do not intend to breastfeed, will be keen to express at least some breast milk for their baby once they understand the importance of this (Spatz 2016). Some mothers may be happy to express their milk but might never want to breastfeed, and it is important for midwives to support mothers in these decisions and support them in whatever level of commitment they feel able to give without judging them (Hurst & Meier 2010).

Activity

Consider what you would say to a mother about the importance of providing breast milk for her baby. Would it be useful to consider breast milk as a medicine? Download and read a journal article about the importance of breast milk for premature babies (for example, Miracle et al 2004).

Expressing milk for premature babies

A mother of a premature infant will need to initiate and maintain lactation until their infant is able to suckle fully at the breast which may not be possible for several weeks or even months. This means that mothers are often feeling anxious about their baby's wellbeing as they make the transition to motherhood and when they are starting to express breast milk. It will therefore be crucial for midwives to provide emotional support as well as information to enable mothers to persevere to achieve their goals. Although having a baby prematurely does not appear to limit mother's ability to produce milk, many of the factors that often occur as part of the overall experience are known to inhibit the production of prolactin, such as maternal complications, tiredness, stress and irregular breast milk expression (Hurst & Meier 2010). The shortened gestation may mean hormones do not reach maximum levels, and lactogenesis II may be delayed which may result in low milk supply in the early days after birth (Arnold 2010).

Mothers should start to express breast milk as soon as possible after birth and should express frequently in the first few days (8 to 10 times daily; Hurst & Meier 2010) with at least one being at night between 2:00 and 6:00 a.m. when prolactin levels are highest (Walker 2017). It may be helpful for mothers to express near the baby or have a photograph or an item of the baby's clothing to help to stimulate oxytocin to enable the milk to flow. The aim should be to produce a milk volume of 750 to 1000 ml a day at the end of the first week to 10 days regardless of the infant's needs at that time (Spatz 2016). This will help to enable mothers to produce an adequate ongoing supply and ultimately to fully breastfeed their baby.

It may be helpful to start by hand expressing and collecting drops of colostrum by syringe from the nipple (UNICEF Baby Friendly Initiative UK 2014), but after this a hospital-grade electric pump is likely to be needed and pumping both breasts at the same time most effective (Renfrew et al 2009). At least 50% of the calories in human milk comes from lipids, and the lipid concentration increases throughout a single milk expression (Spatz 2016). It is therefore important that mothers know this and are encouraged to continue pumping until the flow of milk slows to a few drops, as the last to be expressed will be highest in calories. When expressed milk is stored, the milk fat rises to the top so mothers should be encouraged to gently mix the milk before pouring it into sterile storage containers, otherwise the baby may receive milk with very different calorific content at different feedings (Spatz 2016).

Activity

Based on your knowledge of the physiology of lactation, what suggestions might you make to a mother who is concerned that the volume of milk she is expressing is low? Where and how is expressed breast milk stored in your unit?

Kangaroo care and the effect on milk production

Skin-to-skin or kangaroo care is an important aspect of care for premature infants and documented benefits include: stability of vital signs, increased parent-infant interaction, faster neuro-behavioural maturation, improved sleep patterns (Spatz 2016) and reduced mortality (Conde-Agudelo & Díaz-Rossello 2016). It also provides ready access to the breast and improves milk supply (Conde-Agudelo & Díaz-Rossello 2016; Moore et al 2012) and can mean that the mother is more responsive to her baby's cues. A cohort study in Sweden has demonstrated an association between the amount of time spent providing kangaroo care and breastfeeding in very premature infants (Flacking et al 2011), and evidence from a systematic review suggests that kangaroo care leads to increased duration of breastfeeding of premature infants after discharge home (Renfrew et al 2009). Hake-Brooks and Anderson (2008) in a small study found that kangaroo care increases exclusivity of breast milk feeding at every time point up to 18 months. Kangaroo care has also been shown to decrease the length of hospital stay (Gregson & Blacker 2011).

The transfer of an infant to the mother's chest for kangaroo care can be a stressful event and therefore the duration of kangaroo care should generally be longer than an hour to enable them to settle (Arnold 2010). The baby is placed in a fetal position between the mother's breasts vertically or diagonally with only a nappy and maybe booties and a hat on, covered with a blanket and the mother's clothes. There is no need to limit time spent skin-to-skin unless the mother requests or the baby shows signs of distress (Nyqvist 2013; Spatz 2016). Since 2003 kangaroo care has been recommended as part of high-quality neonatal care (World Health Organization 2003).

Activity

Search the Internet using a phrase such as 'kangaroo care' or 'expecting a premature baby' and look at the information mothers may access. A range of books and DVDs are available to mothers. Consider which of these you feel would be useful to mothers of premature babies you may care for as a midwife.

Mother's experiences

Mothers of premature babies inevitably experience negative and conflicting emotions which are more severe with increasing prematurity (Arnold 2010). The most stressful aspects of neonatal care for a mother of a premature baby are separation and her inability to fully care for her baby (Boucher et al 2011; Flacking et al 2006). Most mothers are separated from their baby as facilities for rooming in are limited. Flacking et al (2006:74) found that this resulted in women feeling like a visitor and 'unimportant to the infant' and that their emotional needs to be close to the infant were not met. Holding their baby with skin-to-skin contact and breastfeeding can be a step towards normalcy and will strengthen the relationship between the mother and baby (Flacking et al 2006). The new UNICEF Baby Friendly Initiative standards (2012) incorporate this at the Stage 3 assessment by including standards that must be met in relation to parent's experiences in the neonatal unit. This includes unrestricted access to their baby, encouragement to touch and respond to their baby and to hold their baby skin-to-skin (UNICEF Baby Friendly Initiative UK 2012). In addition to support from health professionals, mothers may benefit from mother-to-mother support or support from trained peer counsellors who can reduce anxiety and improve breastfeeding outcomes (Spatz 2016).

Activity

Consider what emotional support you would offer to a woman who had given birth to a premature baby if you were the midwife caring for her on the postnatal ward. What support is there for women in the neonatal unit in your place of work? Does this support continue once the baby is at home?

Supporting breastfeeding for a late preterm baby

Late preterm babies, born between 34 and 36 completed weeks of gestation, are not simply smaller than babies born at term but are developmentally different (Walker 2017). They are at greater risk of mortality and morbidity (Dimitriou et al 2010) and have specific needs that can impact on feeding. The last few weeks of gestation are important for growth and development, for example, the brain of a baby born at 36 weeks' gestation weighs 80% of that of a baby born at term (Kinney 2006). Developmental immaturity results in clinical challenges such as: respiratory problems, for example, higher risk of apnoea; temperature instability; higher risk of infection; hyperbilirubinaemia; hypoglycaemia and problems feeding (Dimitriou et al 2010).

Many units in the UK have a transitional care ward where babies with increased needs, such as late preterm babies, can be cared for with their mothers. These units usually have higher ratio of staff to mothers and babies, and this means that more intensive support can be provided. This is likely to be helpful because, as discussed earlier, being fed human milk is especially important for premature babies, but these babies are less likely to be breastfed and, if breastfed, may encounter additional challenges such as higher risk of dehydration (Meier et al 2007).

Late preterm babies are born with fewer stores of subcutaneous and brown fat and therefore have lower energy stores. This is compounded by their inability to feed as well as term babies. Late preterm babies are often sleepy and tire easily when feeding. They have low muscle tone and a weak suck and often find it difficult to coordinate sucking and breathing (Walker 2017). Late preterm babies often feed inefficiently. They may stop feeding before they have taken sufficient volume of milk, particularly as intake of higher volumes of milk are needed which can result in slow weight gain (Walker 2017) and may lead to longer stays in the hospital and/or hospital readmission (Ray & Lorch 2013).

Mothers of late preterm babies may be at risk of delayed lactogenesis II, meaning that they may produce colostrum for a longer period of time. In addition to this, mothers of late preterm babies may not produce as much milk because their babies have a weaker suck and feed for less time which decreases the production of prolactin. Therefore these mothers are likely to need to express breast milk in the same way as mothers of more premature babies (as previously discussed).

There are three main goals in the care of late preterm infants: 1. to reduce the chances of morbidity and poor outcomes, 2. to establish and maintain the mother's milk supply and 3. to ensure the baby has adequate nutritional intake (Walker 2017). To achieve these goals, late preterm babies will need to be fed often to prevent hypoglycaemia and jaundice. As for all babies, the first breastfeed should be within an hour of birth. After this, preterm babies will benefit from being fed hourly for 3 to 4 hours and then every 2 to 3 hours until 12 hours after birth and then at least eight times in 24 hours (Walker 2017). Encouraging mothers to spend as much time as possible in skin-to-skin contact with their baby will reduce the baby's stress levels and help the transition to extra-uterine life and give easy access to the breast (Bergman 2013, Spatz 2016). The midwife should encourage the mother to look for signs that their baby may be ready to feed, such as rapid eye movement under the eyelids, sucking movements and hand-to-mouth movements (Walker 2017). Careful positioning for breastfeeding may be needed – especially if the baby has poor muscle tone – to avoid apnoea and bradycardia. The cradle hold may best be avoided as this may encourage flexion of the baby's neck (Meier et al 2007). If, with frequent cue-based feeding, the baby is not able to obtain enough then expressed colostrum or breast milk can be fed by syringe or cup feeding.

REFLECTION ON THE TRIGGER SCENARIO

Baby Jack was born by caesarean section at 29 weeks' gestation as his mother, Lynne, had pregnancy-induced hypertension. Lynne enjoyed holding Jack against her skin immediately after birth in the operating theatre as he seemed calm and relaxed, although she was amazed at how small he seemed. Lynne is keen to start expressing breast milk for Jack and has asked the midwife what she should do.

Jack will benefit from ongoing skin-to-skin contact with his mother. Despite him being so small, Lynne is confident she can care for him. She is aware that he feels calmer and more settled when she is holding him. She has learned how to hand express and has now expressed some colostrum for Jack; she smiled as the midwife referred to it as *liquid gold*. What information will Lynne need to enable her to establish a good milk supply? What kinds of breast pumps are available in your unit? Would Lynne have unrestricted access to Jack in your unit?

The scenario highlights that Lynne appears to understand the importance of skin-to-skin contact and the benefits of colostrum for her premature baby, Jack. Now that you are familiar with some of the reasons why breast milk is particularly important for premature babies and some of the extra support a mother with a premature baby might need, you should have an insight into how the scenario relates to the evidence. The jigsaw model will now be used to explore the trigger scenario in more depth.

Effective communication

Effective verbal and non-verbal communication will be essential in providing care for Lynne. She may benefit from emotional support to help her cope during this challenging time, and this will mean the midwife will need to be aware when Lynne wants to talk or perhaps when she may not. At times simply being there for her and listening to her concerns may be what is needed. Questions that arise from the scenario might include: Has the midwife caring for Lynne taken time to understand Lynne's concerns about Jack's wellbeing? Is there effective communication between the midwife and staff on the neonatal unit? Has the midwife communicated clearly how important it is that Lynne should start expressing her breast milk and how often she should do this? What has been documented in Lynne's maternity records?

Woman-centred care

Providing care that meets Lynne's individual circumstances and choices is crucial to high-quality maternity care. Questions that arise from the scenario might include: Does Lynne understand the benefits for Jack of caring for him in skin-to-skin contact, providing kangaroo care? Is she keen to do this? Is there anything the midwife can do that would make this more possible for Lynne and Jack? What are Lynne's family circumstances? Does she have support from her partner, members of her family and social network? Might Lynne's partner also be keen to give Jack kangaroo care? When Lynne is fit to go home, will she be easily able to travel to visit Jack?

Using best evidence

There are a number of ways that the midwife caring for Lynne might draw upon best evidence. In addition to evidence about the health effects of feeding breast milk, the midwife would need to be aware of the evidence about how best to support Lynne to optimize her milk supply. This would require understanding of the physiology of lactation and research about the quantity of milk Lynne will need to express in the first week to enable her to produce sufficient breast milk to be able to breastfeed Jack, once he is able to do so. Questions that arise from the scenario might include: How soon would the midwife suggest Lynne starts to express her breast milk? How often would she encourage Lynne to express in the first few days? Why should Lynne express during the night? Evidence is always being updated; how is the midwife keeping her knowledge up to date?

Professional and legal issues

Midwives must always use best evidence in their practice and work in partnership with parents to ensure they deliver care effectively (NMC 2015). Most mothers, once they understand the health-enhancing effects of breast milk for their premature baby, will want to provide some breast milk for their baby even if they do not ultimately intend to breastfeed. Questions that arise from the scenario might include: Has the midwife had a conversation with Lynne to find out if she is fully aware of the benefits of feeding breast milk to Jack? Does Lynne know how to express her breast milk? Has the midwife shown her the equipment and explained how to use it?

Team working

Team working is especially important to provide good care to Lynne and Jack. There will be paediatricians, neonatal nurses and support staff providing care for Jack and obstetricians, midwives and support staff providing care for Lynne. This means that good communication both within these teams and from one team to the other will be needed.

Questions that arise from the scenario might include: Does the midwife caring for Lynne know who is responsible for Jack's care? Have they spoken to each other? Would the midwife be able to visit the neonatal unit with Lynne? Who is responsible for ensuring Lynne has all the information she needs?

Clinical dexterity

As with many aspects of infant feeding, probably the most important skill is good communication. As already discussed, this might involve ensuring Lynne is aware of the importance of providing breast milk for Jack and how often to express to optimize her supply. Therefore an important aspect of communication is the ability to provide clear information about how to express. Initially this might be how to hand express but very quickly Lynne will need to use a breast pump. Often, women expressing for a premature baby are expressing for some time and will benefit from being able to use a double pump to express both breasts at once. Another important skill will be to ensure the breast cups for expressing are the correct size so that they are comfortable and expressing is efficient. Questions that arise from the scenario might include: Has the midwife explained all aspects of how to use a breast pump? How has she ensured that Lynne understands correctly? Has the midwife shown Lynne how and where to wash and sterilize the pump equipment after use?

Models of care

The model of care in many units within the UK would be that, after birth, Jack would be cared for in the neonatal unit and Lynne would be cared for on the postnatal ward. It may be that Lynne will find this upsetting as other mothers would have their babies with them and she will not. This physical separation would also not be conducive to enabling Lynne to start to build a relationship with Jack and may mean that Lynne will need extra emotional support. Questions that arise from the scenario might include: Does Lynne have a named midwife on the postnatal ward? Has the midwife caring for Lynne found out how baby Jack is progressing? How might a close liaison between the midwife caring for Lynne and staff on the neonatal unit be helpful?

Safe environment

The midwife should provide sufficient information and care to maximize safety for both Lynne and Jack. This might, for example, include explaining about safe storage of expressed breast milk. Questions that arise from the scenario might include: Did the midwife explain to Lynne that she should wash her hands before expressing? Where should Lynne store her expressed milk? How should she label this? How long can expressed breast milk be stored in a fridge? How long can expressed breast milk be stored in a freezer? If Jack was to be fed donor breast milk, how would this have been processed to be safe for another baby? Where is your local donor breast milk bank?

Promotes health

Feeding human milk to a premature baby has huge potential to promote health of that infant in the short and long term providing protection against infection, decreased intestinal permeability and increased tolerance of milk feeding. The baby is also less likely to develop NEC and more likely to have good visual acuity and improved neurocognitive performance (Walker 2017). Questions that arise from the scenario might include: How and when might the midwife discuss these health-enhancing effects of breast milk with Lynne? Lynne has chosen to breastfeed, but if she had not, how might the discussion be different? Might the idea of breast milk being like a medicine for a premature baby be helpful in this respect? How can the midwife ensure that these conversations are respectful of each woman's wishes?

Further scenarios

The following scenarios enable you to consider how specific situations influence the care the midwife provides. Use the jigsaw model to explore the issues raised in each situation.

SCENARIO 1

Fatima gave birth to her baby boy, Raffiel, at 32 weeks' gestation. He is being cared for in the neonatal unit and is making good progress. Fatima is about to go home from the postnatal ward and will be returning to visit every day. She is expressing breast milk for Raffiel but is concerned that she may not have as much time to express her milk. She asks the midwife on the postnatal ward a number of questions as she prepares to go home.

Practice point

Although Fatima may be looking forward to going home, she is likely to feel even more separated from baby Raffiel who is not yet ready to go home from the neonatal unit. Continuing to receive breast milk will enhance Raffiel's health and wellbeing into the future, so this is an important aspect of the care Fatima can provide for him. Once she goes home, Fatima may get mixed messages about breastfeeding from members of her family and social network.

Further points specific to Scenario 1 include:

1. How can the midwife provide emotional support for Fatima as she prepares to go home and is concerned about being even more separated from Raffiel?
2. What suggestions might the midwife make to help Fatima maintain her supply of breast milk?
3. Might some agreed short-term goals help Fatima to remain motivated to express her milk?
4. When Fatima visits Raffiel, why will kangaroo care be important to both of them?
5. Does Fatima have a hospital-grade breast pump available to her at home?
6. Why might a pump that enables her to express both breasts at once be helpful for Fatima?
7. Does Fatima have sufficient bottles or other suitable containers to take with her for breast milk expression, and is she clear how these should be labelled?
8. Does Fatima know how expressed breast milk should be stored?

SCENARIO 2

Baby Miles was born at around 36 weeks' gestation. He is breastfeeding fairly well but his mother Fiona is worried because he is rather sleepy and occasionally slips off her breast whilst he is feeding.

Practice point

Mothers of late preterm babies need extra support to feed their babies. Even though these babies may appear like smaller term babies, they are vulnerable to a range of poor outcomes and may not take enough milk for their needs.

Further points specific to Scenario 2 include:

1. What cues should Fiona look for to maximize opportunities for feeding Miles?
2. Late preterm babies need to feed often initially as otherwise they are unlikely to take sufficient milk. How often would the midwife suggest Fiona feeds Miles in the first 24 hours?
3. What positions might be most helpful for Fiona to hold Miles for breastfeeding?

4. Why would plenty of skin-to-skin contact be helpful?
5. Is Fiona likely to need to express any breast milk? If so, how might she start to do this?
6. If Fiona is expressing breast milk and feeding Miles, when should she do this in relation to his feeds?
7. How does the fat content of a breast milk change throughout each feed?

Conclusion

Having a premature baby is a very stressful life event for women and families. Providing good support can make a real difference to both how women feel and to their ability to supply breast milk for their baby. Midwives have a key role to play in ensuring that women have correct evidence-based information to enable them to make important infant-feeding choices, emotional support to help them to cope and practical support to help them learn the skill of milk expression.

Resources

Best Beginnings. *Small wonders film clips.* Available at: https://www.bestbeginnings .org.uk/small-wonders.

Bliss for babies born premature or sick. Available at: https://www.bliss.org.uk/.

Kangaroo mother care: support for parents and staff of premature babies. Available at: http://www.kangaroomothercare.com/home.aspx.

The Breastfeeding Network. *Expressing and soring breast milk.* Available at: https:// www.breastfeedingnetwork.org.uk/wp-content/pdfs/BFNExpressing_and_ Storing.pdf. U

United Kingdom Association for Milk Banking. *'Every drop counts'.* Available at: http://www.ukamb.org/.

References

Arnold, L.D.W., 2010. Human Milk in the NICU: Policy Into Practice. Jones and Bartlett, London.

Bergman, N., 2013. Breastfeeding and perinatal neuroscience. In: Watson Genna, C. (Ed.), Supporting Sucking Skills in Breastfeeding Infants, second ed. Jones and Bartlett, Burlington.

Boucher, C.A., Brazal, P.M., Graham-Certosini, C., et al., 2011. Mothers' breastfeeding experiences in the NICU. Neonatal Netw. 30, 21–28.

Conde-Agudelo, A., Díaz-Rossello, J.L., 2016. Kangaroo mother care to reduce morbidity and mortality in low birthweight infants. Cochrane Database Syst. Rev. (8), Art No. CD002771, doi:10.1002/14651858.CD002771.pub4.

Dimitriou, G., Fouzas, S., Georgakis, V., et al., 2010. Determinants of morbidity in late preterm infants. Early Hum. Dev. 86, 587–591.

Flacking, R., Ewald, U., Nyqvist, K.H., Starrin, B., 2006. Trustful bonds: a key to "becoming a mother" and to reciprocal breastfeeding. Stories of mothers of very preterm infants at a neonatal unit. Soc. Sci. Med. 62, 70–80.

Flacking, R., Ewald, U., Wallin, L., 2011. Positive effect of kangaroo mother care on long-term breastfeeding in very preterm infants. J. Obstet. Gynecol. Neonatal Nurs. 40, 190–197.

Gregson, S., Blacker, J., 2011. Kangaroo care in pre-term or low birth weight babies in a postnatal ward. Br. J. Midwifery 19, 568–577.

Hake-Brooks, S.J., Anderson, G.C., 2008. Kangaroo care and breastfeeding of mother-preterm infant dyads 0-18 months: a randomized, controlled trial. Neonatal Netw. 27, 151–159.

Hurst, N., Meier, P., 2010. Breastfeeding the preterm infant. In: Riordan, J., Wambach, K. (Eds.), Breastfeeding and Lactation. Jones and Bartlett, Burlington.

Kimak, K.S., de Castro Antunes, M.M., Braga, T.D., et al., 2015. Influence of enteral nutrition on occurrences of necrotizing enterocolitis in very-low-birth-weight infants. J. Pediatr. Gastroenterol. Nutr. 61, 445–450.

Kinney, H.C., 2006. The near-term (late preterm) human brain and risk for periventricular leukomalacia: a review. Semin. Perinatol. 30, 81–88.

Lucas, A., Cole, T.J., 1990. Breast milk and neonatal necrotising enterocolitis. Lancet 336, 1519–1523.

McGuire, W., Anthony, M.Y., 2003. Donor human milk versus formula for preventing necrotising enterocolitis in preterm infants: systematic review. Arch. Dis. Child. Fetal Neonatal Ed. 88, F11–F14.

Meier, P.P., Furman, L.M., Degenhardt, M., 2007. Increased lactation risk for late preterm infants and mothers: evidence and management strategies to protect breastfeeding. J. Midwifery Womens Health 52, 579–587.

Miracle, D.J., Meier, P.P., Bennett, P.A., 2004. Mothers' decisions to change from formula to mothers' milk for very-low-birth-weight infants. J. Obstet. Gynecol. Neonatal Nurs. 33, 692–703.

Moore, E.R., Anderson, G.C., Bergman, N., Dowswell, T., 2012. Early skin-to-skin contact for mothers and their healthy newborn infants. Cochrane Database Syst. Rev. (5), Art. No.: CD003519, doi:10.1002/14651858.CD003519 .pub3.

NMC, 2015. The Code: Professional Standards of Practice and Behaviour for Nurses and Midwives. Nursing and Midwifery Council., London. Available at: https:// www.nmc.org.uk/globalassets/sitedocuments/nmc-publications/nmc-code.pdf.

Nyqvist, K.H., 2013. Breastfeeding preterm infants. In: Genna, C.W. (Ed.), Supporting Suckling Skills in Breastfeeding Infants. Jones and Bartlett, London.

Quigley, M.A., Hockley, C., Carson, C., et al., 2012. Breastfeeding is associated with improved child cognitive development: a population-based cohort study. J. Pediatr. 160, 25–32.

Ray, K.N., Lorch, S.A., 2013. Hospitalization of early preterm, late preterm, and term infants during the first year of life by gestational age. Hosp. Pediatr. 3, 194–203.

Renfrew, M.J., Craig, D., Dyson, L., et al., 2009. Breastfeeding promotion for infants in neonatal units: a systematic review and economic analysis. Health Technol. Assess. 13, 1–146, iii-iv. doi:10.3310/hta13400.

Spatz, D.L., 2016. The use of human milk and breastfeeding in the neonatal intensive care unit. In: Wambach, K., Riordan, J. (Eds.), Breastfeeding and Human Lactation, fifth ed. Jones and Bartlett Learning, Burlington.

UNICEF Baby Friendly Initiative UK, 2012. Guide to the Baby Friendly Initiative Standards. UNICEF Baby Friendly Initiative UK., London.

UNICEF Baby Friendly Initiative UK, 2014. The UNICEF UK Baby Friendly Initiative Train the Trainer. UNICEF Baby Friendly Initiative UK, London.

Vohr, B.R., Poindexter, B.B., Dusick, A.M., et al. & NICHD Neonatal Research Network, 2006. Beneficial effects of breast milk in the neonatal intensive care unit on the developmental outcome of extremely low birth weight infants at 18 months of age. Pediatrics 18, e115–e123.

Walker, M., 2017. Breastfeeding Management for the Clinician: Using the Evidence, fourth ed. Jones and Bartlett, Burlington.

World Health Organization, 2003. Kangaroo Mother Care: A Practical Guide. World Health Organization, Geneva.

CHAPTER 12

Breastfeeding mothers, their family, community and the wider societal context

TRIGGER SCENARIO

Danielle is a 25-year-old woman who has recently had her second baby, Lily. She intends to breastfeed Lily for 6 months until she returns to work just as she did her son, Joshua. When Danielle chose to breastfeed Joshua she was the first in her family to do so. She said, 'I felt a bit embarrassed with him because I kept thinking nobody else has done it.' She was persuaded to breastfeed by her partner, Ethan, whose family had all breastfed but then found it convenient and straightforward and decided to continue. Her neighbour also breastfed and Danielle explained, 'I was encouraged by her as well. We experienced it together.' She also felt supported by her sister-in-law who was breastfeeding her child who was the same age as Joshua.

Introduction

The social, cultural and political context within which mothers feed their babies shapes their decisions and experiences in many ways. Breastfeeding is a personal activity, but at the same time, it is a public concern that is affected by societal values, cultures and norms. Women breastfeed their babies within family and social networks, and the responses of people close to them can affect their emotions, attitudes and consequently behaviour (Marshall & Godfrey 2012). Therefore midwives supporting women to breastfeed will need to consider ways of helping women to harness sources of support from within their family and wider social networks and to develop ways to manage negative and unhelpful comments or actions that could undermine their breastfeeding.

Attitudes towards infant feeding are shaped unconsciously from a young age; for example, a child seeing their own mother breastfeed a younger sibling can mean that breastfeeding becomes seen as the normal way to feed a baby. Mothers who have seen a relative breastfeed and viewed this positively are more likely to choose to breastfeed and feel confident about this (Hoddinott & Pill 1999). Conversely, when young children are given baby dolls that bottle feed and/or they see mothers bottle feeding babies, then bottle feeding is more likely to be seen as the norm.

Having made the decision to breastfeed, many women stop before they want to do so. The reasons for stopping highlighted within the Infant Feeding Survey include technical aspects such as painful breasts and the baby not taking the breast and suckling effectively (McAndrew et al 2012) which could be resolved by providing more support in the early days of breastfeeding. Another key reason women stop breastfeeding is when their baby is feeding frequently and mothers believe they have insufficient milk (McAndrew et al 2012), and this may be influenced by negative comments from significant people within mothers' family and social networks.

Mothers who are older (30 years and over), who are from managerial and professional occupations, left full-time education when they were over 18 years or who live in the least-deprived areas are most likely to start to breastfeed and continue for longer (McAndrew et al 2012). It would therefore seem appropriate for healthcare providers such as midwives to provide more support to those least likely to continue to breastfeed. However, those in most need of support, such as younger women living in deprived areas, are least likely to engage with health services. This has been called the *inverse care law* (Tudor Hart 1971) and can potentially increase existing health inequalities.

Some of the challenges women encounter as they start their breastfeeding journey have been discussed in Chapter 6 with consideration of the social and cultural context within which these occur. In this chapter, the broader family, community and societal context is considered in more detail. This includes discussion of the contribution of significant people within mothers' family such as fathers, sources of support at the community level such as breastfeeding peer supporters and consideration of some of the challenges women may encounter when breastfeeding in public places.

UNICEF Baby Friendly Maternity standards

The following are the maternity standards that are most relevant to this chapter:

- Support pregnant women to recognize the importance of breastfeeding and early relationships for the health and wellbeing of their baby
- Support mothers to make informed decisions regarding the introduction of food or fluids other than breast milk

Fathers

The baby's father often has most influence on the mother's decisions about infant feeding (Rempel et al 2016) and therefore fathers have a vital role to play in supporting their breastfeeding partner. Many fathers want their baby to be breastfed and believe this to be the healthiest choice for their partner and baby; however, some fathers do not feel it is their choice to make (Mitchell-Box & Braun 2012). Fathers respond in different ways to having a new baby and to breastfeeding, and they can sometimes feel as if they are on the periphery when most attention is focused on the mother and infant (Wambach 2016). It is therefore important to involve them in conversations about infant feeding as not doing so may emphasize feelings of inadequacy. Early involvement can also help fathers to strengthen their relationship and bond with their baby.

Educational interventions for fathers have been found to be effective to increase breastfeeding initiation and exclusivity (Mitchell-Box & Braun 2013). These may start antenatally in preparation for parenting sessions. Brown and Davies (2014) found that fathers wanted to feel included and wanted specific information about how they could support their partner, particularly when problems with breastfeeding occurred. Transition to fatherhood can be stressful and place strain on the couple's relationship, and fathers can sometimes feel left out and be jealous of the closeness between mother and baby (Brown & Davies 2014). Meeting other fathers might be helpful to share experiences to resolve some of these issues, and support groups for fathers exist in some areas.

Sometimes fathers are very keen to bottle feed their baby as they may feel that this is the only way to achieve closeness and bonding (Wambach 2016). This can lead to mothers expressing breast milk as soon as possible to facilitate this, which ultimately may not be helpful to encourage continued exclusive breastfeeding. There are many other ways that a father may be able to interact with their baby, for example, by giving the baby a massage, bathing or cuddling the baby. In a randomized controlled trial in Canada, a co-parenting breastfeeding support intervention in which parents were encouraged to work together to achieve their parenting goals was found to increase breastfeeding rates, father's confidence in breastfeeding and mother's satisfaction with fathers' involvement with breastfeeding (Abbass-Dick et al 2015).

Activity

When you next meet a father in clinical practice, ask him about his views about parenting and childcare. Are you aware of sessions available to fathers only in your area of work? If not, use the Internet and ask community contacts to enable you to make a list that you could use in practice.

Family-centred breastfeeding care

The influence of significant people within a mother's family and immediate social network is an important consideration for midwives and others caring for breastfeeding women. Family and significant others within a mother's social circle are often broadly considered to be supportive of mothers with newborn babies, but this can either work to encourage or discourage breastfeeding or sometimes both at different times. For example, if a mother is breastfeeding within a family where bottle feeding is the norm, casual comments about how often a baby is feeding is likely to undermine a mother's confidence and self-efficacy and encourage her to believe that she does not have enough milk for her baby (Marshall et al 2007).

Grandmothers of the new baby are generally considered to influence a mother's decisions about baby care and infant feeding, and this is supported by a systematic review of 13 quantitative studies from a range of countries (but not the UK) that found that grandmothers can influence exclusive breastfeeding (Negin et al 2016). Although new mothers often need and want support from grandmothers, because grandmothers bring their beliefs about infant feeding to this support, it is not always conducive to continued or exclusive breastfeeding (Grassley & Eschiti 2008). This may depend on the kind of support that is provided by the grandmother. An analysis of data from the Millennium cohort study found that mothers with more frequent contact with grandmothers (either maternal or paternal) were less likely to choose to breastfeed and were likely to breastfeed for a shorter time. The authors suggest that this could be because, when more practical support is provided and grandmothers take a greater part in childcare including infant feeding, this discourages breastfeeding (Emmott & Mace 2015). This study also found this to be the case for parenting involvement from fathers, but interestingly the father's presence, perhaps capturing emotional support, encouraged breastfeeding initiation (Emmott & Mace 2015). This is also reinforced by a more recent study that found that, when fathers were more involved and appreciative of breastfeeding per se, this could be associated with less breastfeeding; however, when fathers were responsive and sensitive to the mother's needs, this was associated with increased breastfeeding (Rempel et al 2016).

A study conducted in Scotland highlighted that parents having their first baby often experience a mismatch between their expectations and the reality of how they might receive practical and emotional support from family, friends and health professionals (Hoddinott et al 2012). Mothers in this study did not generally feel able to ask for help, leading the authors to conclude that significant people in mothers' close social circle should be involved in discussions about parenting and breastfeeding and that help should be offered proactively (Hoddinott et al 2012).

Activity

Consider the range of sessions that aim to prepare parents for parenting available in your area of work, and think about ways that family members might be involved more in discussions about parenting and breastfeeding.

Peer support

Women may also receive support from peers. Peer support for breastfeeding mothers is usually a combination of emotional, practical and informational support provided by someone from a similar background or area and who has breastfed themselves (McFadden et al 2017). Peer supporters are therefore mothers who have experience of breastfeeding and are trained to provide support to other mothers. They are often from the same community as the mothers they support and may share characteristics such as socio-economic status, ethnicity and language so that they can provide assistance to a mother that is culturally and socially appropriate. Peer support in the UK is provided by a range of organizations such as the National Childbirth Trust (NCT), Breastfeeding Network (BfN), Association of Breastfeeding Mothers, La Leche League, local peer support organizations and is commissioned by some NHS trusts and local authorities. Peer support can be either voluntary or provided by paid workers.

Breastfeeding peer support can be provided in a variety of ways. It can be offered as a structured organized programme that starts during pregnancy and continues throughout women's feeding experience or can be accessed by mothers when they feel they need support. It can be provided within groups or to individual mothers or a combination of both. It is sometimes provided as part of more general support to new mothers or may be feeding specific. Peer support can be offered face-to-face in a range of settings, such as hospital postnatal wards, the woman's own home and/or community centres. It can also be provided by telephone, text messaging and via social media (Thomson et al 2015).

A Cochrane review of healthy mothers and babies found that any support, whether from health professionals or peers, is beneficial to help mothers to breastfeed more exclusively and for longer. However, a systematic review of randomized controlled trials specifically focusing on peer support did not find a significant effect in studies conducted in the UK (Jolly et al 2012). The authors suggest that this is likely to be because mothers in the UK already receive postnatal care from midwives for the first 10 days and thereafter see health visitors who can provide support for breastfeeding, and therefore the addition of low-intensity peer support was not found to be effective. However, this does not mean that all women do not find peer support helpful. It may be that peer support is helpful to some women in some circumstances but not to others. For example, a qualitative study carried out in the northwest of England found that women felt that peer supporters helped them to reach their breastfeeding goals (Thomson et al 2012). It also may be that women choose not to access peer support. A qualitative study conducted in Cornwall found that women did not attend peer support groups because they expected their infant-feeding decisions to be judged (Hunt & Thomson 2016).

Breastfeeding in public places

Women who continue to breastfeed will usually want to feed their baby outside their home, and whilst this does not worry some mothers, for others it can be challenging. Although many women do feed in public places, most prefer a quiet place to sit or to use a mother and baby room. In the infant feeding survey, around half of the women who said they breastfed in public had encountered problems in doing so, such as finding somewhere suitable, and a few mothers had been stopped from breastfeeding or been made to feel uncomfortable whilst breastfeeding (McAndrew et al 2012).

In the UK since 2010, women who are breastfeeding have been protected from discrimination by the Equality Act. The legislation varies across countries within the UK. In Scotland, there has been protection for longer through the Breastfeeding etc. (Scotland) Act which has been in place since 2005. This makes it an offence to stop or prevent infant feeding in a public place for a child under 2 years old. In Northern Ireland, the Sex Discrimination (Northern Ireland) Order 1976 was amended in 2008 making it illegal to discriminate against women who have recently given birth (within the last 26 weeks). However, protection from discrimination is only part of this as women often feel uncomfortable breastfeeding in public places because of sexualization of breasts and the bottle-feeding culture within the UK. Women are also sometimes constrained by the views and beliefs of their partners who may not be happy for them to feed in public places.

Breastfeeding and return to work

Many mothers want to continue to breastfeed after they return to work but do not commonly do so. The length of maternity leave in the UK has been extended in recent years and perhaps unsurprisingly mothers are returning to work later and many return to part-time work (McAndrew et al 2012). Parents can also apply for shared parental leave. If a breastfeeding woman returns to work, her employer has an obligation to provide facilities for her to do so. Employers should have a policy to support breastfeeding mothers; they should enable a breastfeeding mother to take flexible breaks, provide a suitable space for expressing and a fridge to store breast milk. The mother should write a letter to her employer informing them of her return to work and her wish to continue breastfeeding. The employer will then need to carry out a risk assessment to ensure her health and safety at work.

REFLECTION ON THE TRIGGER SCENARIO

Danielle is a 25-year-old woman who has recently had her second baby, Lily. She intends to breastfeed Lily for 6 months until she returns to work just as she did her son, Joshua. When Danielle chose to breastfeed Joshua she was the first in her family to do so. She said, 'I felt a bit embarrassed with him because I kept thinking nobody else has done it.' She was persuaded to breastfeed by her partner, Ethan, whose family had all breastfed but then found it convenient and straightforward and decided to continue. Her neighbour also breastfed and Danielle explained, 'I was encouraged by her as well. We experienced it together.' She also felt supported by her sister-in-law who was breastfeeding her child who was the same age as Joshua.

Once she started breastfeeding, Danielle found this much easier and more convenient than 'all that sterilizing'. This scenario is based on a situation encountered in clinical practice as part of a research study (with all names changed). It demonstrates how a woman's previous exposure to breastfeeding can affect her intentions but also how this can be modified when, for people close to her, breastfeeding is seen to be the normal way to feed a baby as was the case for Danielle's partner. This is likely to have been reinforced as Danielle continued to breastfeed as both her neighbour and sister-in-law were also breastfeeding babies of a similar age.

The scenario highlights that, although Danielle was initially ambivalent about breastfeeding, she was influenced by significant people within her social network and eventually chose to breastfeed both her children. Now that you are familiar with some of the evidence that underpins the ways that key people within mothers' social networks can influence their decision to start and continue to breastfeed, you should have an insight into how the scenario relates to the evidence. The jigsaw model will now be used to explore the trigger scenario in more depth.

Effective communication

The key to effective communication for health professionals providing care for Danielle is likely to be to build on her existing knowledge and resources available to her for parenting and as part of this breastfeeding. This would enable identification of any gaps and is more likely to meet her emotional needs. An approach that prioritizes breastfeeding rather than paying attention to Danielle's emotional needs as a parent more generally may be perceived as pressure rather than support. Questions that arise from the scenario might include: How might the care provided by the community midwife and health visitor add to the support provided by members of her family and social network? What questions might the midwife ask Danielle? What type of questions might these be? Why is listening actively to Danielle's experiences likely to be important to providing care for her and her family?

Woman-centred care

To provide good woman-centred care, it is essential to involve members of Danielle's family in discussions about parenting, and this is likely to include infant feeding. Questions that arise from the scenario might include: How might the midwife involve Ethan in the care provided for Danielle? Might it have been helpful for Ethan to attend preparation for parenting sessions before Lily was born? Is peer support available in Danielle's local area? How might the community midwife discuss peer support with Danielle? Might Danielle benefit from considering ways to manage comments from her mother who has bottle fed all of her babies?

Using best evidence

There is a paucity of good quality evidence to inform health professionals and others about the nature of psychosocial care and support that may be most helpful to enable mothers to breastfeed their babies. The nature of this support may depend on the cultural and social context within which the family lives and can be detrimental or helpful to breastfeeding mothers to reach their goals. It seems that an approach that involves other family members and is coordinated, sensitive and responsive to a mother's needs is most likely to be helpful for mothers and more effective in terms of sustaining breastfeeding (Rempel et al 2016). Questions that arise from the scenario might include: How might the community midwife start to encourage such an approach? Would it be helpful to start to work towards this during pregnancy? How might this be continued in the early days after Lily's birth?

Professional and legal issues

Midwives should ensure that the needs of women and their families are recognized and care delivered effectively by working in partnership with them (NMC 2015). Questions that arise from the scenario might include:

How might the midwife ensure her knowledge about effective support for parenting and infant feeding from women's family and social network is up to date? Working in partnership with a mother and her family is likely to empower her to use appropriate support from her social network; how might the community midwife do this? Is infant feeding likely to be Danielle's primary concern?

Team working

The most important team working for the community midwife will be working with Danielle's family. In addition to this, liaison with the health visitor to ensure a smooth transition of care will be important. It will also be helpful for the community midwife to work closely with local peer support organizations to ensure care provided is complementary rather than conflicting. Questions that arise from the scenario might include: Do the community midwives have a good working relationship with the health visitors? Is the midwife aware of the opportunities for peer support locally? Who might be involved in delivering preparation for parenting sessions? Do these continue after the birth of the baby?

Clinical dexterity

Communication skills are likely to be the most important clinical skill in caring for Danielle and her family. Sensitive, family-centred care within which the midwife actively listens to parents' wishes and concerns and respecting their decisions, even if these may be counter to their own beliefs, will be crucial. Questions that arise from the scenario might include: What care might Danielle expect from the community midwife? How might the midwife provide evidence-based information without Danielle feeling pressure to continue to breastfeed? What kinds of conversation might Danielle find most helpful?

Models of care

A model of care that provides continuity during pregnancy and after the birth of the baby is most likely to enable the midwife to build a relationship with Danielle and other members of her family. This would be likely to help them to build a relationship of trust that may enable Danielle to ask for help if needed. Questions that arise from the scenario might include: Does Danielle have a named community midwife? What might the midwife have discussed with Danielle when she was pregnant with Joshua? As Danielle had breastfed Joshua previously, how might this conversation have been different when she was pregnant with Lily?

Safe environment

If a breastfeeding woman returns to work, it is important that the employer carries out a risk assessment, and there must be facilities for safe storage of breast milk. Questions that arise from the scenario might include: When might be an appropriate time to have a conversation with Danielle about the possibility of expressing breast milk on her return to work? Is she aware of her rights? Are there any useful video clips that would provide helpful information to her about expressing breast milk and return to work? Is Danielle aware of how long breast milk can be stored in the fridge and in the freezer?

Promotes health

The midwife has a key role to play in promoting the emotional health of mothers within their family and social context. Maximizing opportunities to engage family members in discussions about infant feeding are likely to help with this. Questions that arise from the scenario might include: How can the midwife demonstrate respect for Danielle's infant feeding choices? What resources might the midwife provide or suggest Danielle might access?

Further scenarios

The following scenarios enable you to consider how specific situations influence the care the midwife provides. Use the jigsaw model to explore the issues raised in each situation.

SCENARIO 1

Amelia is a 29-year-old solicitor who is breastfeeding her first baby, Hayley. Although she has chosen to breastfeed, she is not sure how long she will continue to do so. When the community midwife visits, Amelia tells her that Hayley is having a formula feeding each evening so that her husband can feed her.

Practice point

Fathers often want to feed their baby, and many women like Amelia will introduce a formula feed to enable this to happen. In this situation, it is important to take care to acknowledge Amelia's choice whilst at the same time ensuring she understands the effect that this will have on her ongoing milk supply.

Further points specific to Scenario 1 include:

1. What communication skills will the midwife need in this discussion?
2. Open questions are most likely to enable the midwife to understand Amelia's decision-making process most thoroughly. What question might she ask?
3. Would it be helpful to involve Amelia's partner in this discussion if possible?
4. What activities other than feeding could enable Amelia's husband to interact fully with Hayley?
5. What factor in the breast milk will reduce Amelia's breast milk supply if her breasts become over full?
6. What changes will occur in Hayley's gut from having a formula feed?

SCENARIO 2

Gillian has been breastfeeding her baby, George, since birth with few problems. Her mother and aunt live nearby; both breastfed their children, and they have been providing practical help, such as cooking dinner for her. Before she became pregnant, Gillian was studying photography at college and is keen to return to the course. She asks the midwife what she will need to do to be able to return to her studies and continue to breastfeed.

Practice point

Expressing breast milk whilst returning to work or studies can be a challenge for some women, but providing relevant information and ensuring they know their rights and the law will enable them the choice to do so if they wish.

Further points specific to Scenario 2 include:

1. What will the college need to provide for Gillian?
2. What will Gillian need to know about expressing and storing breast milk?
3. What kind of bag will Gillian need to transfer her breast milk from college to home?
4. Are there childcare facilities at the college available to Gillian so that she can breastfeed George rather than express?
5. How often might Gillian need to express throughout the day when at college?
6. How should Gillian defrost her breast milk when a carer will be feeding George?

Conclusion

The family and social context within which women feed their baby has considerable impact on their decisions and experiences. The midwife has an important role in preparing women to meet some of the challenges they may encounter and helping women to harness support from those close to them and from the community where they live.

Resources

BfN leaflet on expressing and storage of breast milk. Available at: https://www.breastfeedingnetwork.org.uk/wpcontent/pdfs/BFNExpressing_and_Storing.pdf.

Fatherhood Institute. Available at: http://www.fatherhoodinstitute.org/2016/bringing-fathers-in-resources-for-advocates-practitioners-and-researchers/.

La Leche League. Available at: https://www.laleche.org.uk/.

McFadden, A., Gavine, A., Renfrew, M.J., et al., 2017. Support for healthy breastfeeding mothers with healthy term babies. Cochrane Database Syst. Rev. (2), Art. No.: CD001141, doi:10.1002/14651858.CD001141.pub5.

NCT. Available at: https://www.nct.org.uk/parenting.

NICE PN guideline. Available at: https://www.nice.org.uk/guidance/cg37/resources/postnatal-care-up-to-8-weeks-after-birth-975391596997.

References

Abbass-Dick, J., Stern, S.B., Nelson, L.E., et al., 2015. Coparenting breastfeeding support and exclusive breastfeeding: a randomized controlled trial. Pediatrics 135, 102–110.

Brown, A., Davies, R., 2014. Fathers' experiences of supporting breastfeeding: challenges for breastfeeding promotion and education. Maternal & Child Nutrition 10, 510–526.

Emmott, E.H., Mace, R., 2015. Practical support from fathers and grandmothers is associated with lower levels of breastfeeding in the UK Millennium Cohort Study. PLoS ONE 10, e0133547.

Grassley, J., Eschiti, V., 2008. Grandmother breastfeeding support: what do mothers need and want? Birth 35, 329–335.

Hoddinott, P., Craig, L.C.A., Britten, J., McInnes, R.M., 2012. A serial qualitative interview study of infant feeding experiences: idealism meets realism. BMJ Open 14, e000504. doi:10.1136/bmjopen-2011-000504.

Hoddinott, P., Pill, R., 1999. Qualitative study of decisions about infant feeding among women in east end of London. BMJ 318, 30–34.

Hunt, L., Thomson, G., 2016. Pressure and judgement within a dichotomous landscape of infant feeding: a grounded theory study to explore why breastfeeding women do not access peer support provision. Maternal & Child Nutrition doi:10.1111/mcn.12279. [Epub ahead of print].

Jolly, K., Ingram, L., Khan, K.S., et al., 2012. Systematic review of peer support for breastfeeding continuation: metaregression analysis of the effect of setting, intensity, and timing. BMJ 344, d8287. doi:10.1136/bmj.d8287.

Marshall, J., Godfrey, M., 2012. Shifting identities: social and cultural factors that shape decision-making around breastfeeding. In: Liamputtong, P. (Ed.), Infant Feeding Practices: A Cross Cultural Perspective. Springer, New York.

Marshall, J.L., Godfrey, M., Renfrew, M.J., 2007. Being a 'good mother': Managing breastfeeding and merging identities. Social Science & Medicine 65, 2147–2159.

McAndrew, F., Thompson, J., Fellows, L., et al., 2012. Infant Feeding Survey 2010. Health and Social Care Information Centre, London.

McFadden, A., Gavine, A., Renfrew, M.J., et al., 2017. Support for healthy breastfeeding mothers with healthy term babies. Cochrane Database Syst. Rev. (2), Art. No.: CD001141, doi:10.1002/14651858.CD001141.pub5.

Mitchell-Box, K.M., Braun, K.L., 2012. Fathers' thoughts on breastfeeding and implications for a theory-based intervention. J. Obstet. Gynecol. Neonatal Nurs. 41, E41–E50.

Mitchell-Box, K.M., Braun, K.L., 2013. Impact of male-partner-focused interventions on breastfeeding initiation, exclusivity, and continuation. J. Hum. Lact. 29, 473–479.

National Institute for Health and Care Excellence (NICE), 2006, updated 2015. Postnatal care up to 8 weeks after birth. NICE CG37. https://www.nice.org.uk/guidance/cg37.

Negin, J., Coffman, J., Vizintin, P., Raynes-Greenow, C., 2016. The influence of grandmothers on breastfeeding rates: a systematic review. BMC Pregnancy Childbirth 16, 91.

NMC, 2015. The Code: Professional Standards of Practice and Behaviour for Nurses and Midwives. Nursing and Midwifery Council., London. Available at: https://www.nmc.org.uk/globalassets/sitedocuments/nmc-publications/nmc-code.pdf.

Rempel, L.A., Rempel, J.K., Moore, K.C.J., 2016. Relationships between types of father breastfeeding support and breastfeeding outcomes. Matern Child Nutr. doi:10.1111/mcn.12337. [Epub ahead of print].

Thomson, G., Balaam, M.-C., Hymers, K., 2015. Building social capital through breastfeeding peer support: insights from an evaluation of a voluntary breastfeeding peer support service in northwest England. Int. Breastfeed. J. 10, 15.

Thomson, G., Crossland, N., Dykes, F., 2012. Giving me hope: women's reflections on a breastfeeding peer support service. Matern. Child Nutr. 8, 340–353.

Tudor Hart, J., 1971. The inverse care law. Lancet 297, 405–412.

Wambach, K., 2016. The familial and social context of breastfeeding. In: Wambach, K., Riordan, J. (Eds.), Breastfeeding and Human Lactation. Jones and Bartlett, Burlington.

Page numbers followed by "*f*" indicate figures, "*t*" indicate tables, and "*b*" indicate boxes.